# The Affordable Care Act and Integrated Behavioral Health Care

This book provides a scholarly discussion of arguably the most important advance in U.S. public health services since Medicare 50 years ago – how the Federal program known as the Patient Care and Affordable Care Act of 2010 (ACA) or "Obamacare" became law. It addresses ACA in terms of its impact on improving health and behavioral health services for key diverse populations in America, including people with disabilities, consumers, women, racial and ethnic minorities, and veterans and their families.

From the very beginning, ACA was controversial and the topic of heated political debate at both state and national levels. This book examines more closely how the legislation was developed, including the political history of the act; the many advocacy efforts at the national level and the community-based action strategies at the grassroots level; how ACA will affect a broad cross-section of America; the integration of health and behavioral health services as a key component of ACA; the financing of ACA and parity for behavioral health services.

This book was originally published as a special issue of the *Journal of Social Work in Disability & Rehabilitation*.

**Dr. Ford H. Kuramoto**, LCSW has over 30 years of experience in public health research and policy and health and behavioral health services integration field. He worked and consulted with NIMH, UCLA School of Medicine, White House National Drug Control Policy, and SAMHSA. He is the President of Magna Systems, Incorporated.

**Dr. Francis K. Yuen** is a Social Work Professor at California State University, Sacramento, USA. He has published widely and served as the editor for the *Journal of Social Work in Disability & Rehabilitation* since 2003. He has been a principal investigator, evaluator, and trainer for national and local service organizations.

# The Affordable Care Act and Integrated Behavioral Health Care

Meeting the health and behavioral health needs of a diverse society

**Edited by**
Ford H. Kuramoto and
Francis K. Yuen

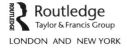

LONDON AND NEW YORK

First published 2015
by Routledge
2 Park Square, Milton Park, Abingdon, Oxon, OX14 4RN, UK

and by Routledge
711 Third Avenue, New York, NY 10017, USA

*Routledge is an imprint of the Taylor & Francis Group, an informa business*

© 2015 Taylor & Francis

All rights reserved. No part of this book may be reprinted or reproduced
or utilised in any form or by any electronic, mechanical, or other means,
now known or hereafter invented, including photocopying and recording,
or in any information storage or retrieval system, without permission in
writing from the publishers.

*Trademark notice*: Product or corporate names may be trademarks or
registered trademarks, and are used only for identification and
explanation without intent to infringe.

*British Library Cataloguing in Publication Data*
A catalogue record for this book is available from the British Library

ISBN 13: 978-1-138-84876-4

Typeset in ITC Garamond
by RefineCatch Limited, Bungay, Suffolk

**Publisher's Note**
The publisher accepts responsibility for any inconsistencies that may have
arisen during the conversion of this book from journal articles to book chapters,
namely the possible inclusion of journal terminology.

**Disclaimer**
Every effort has been made to contact copyright holders for their permission to
reprint material in this book. The publishers would be grateful to hear from any
copyright holder who is not here acknowledged and will undertake to rectify
any errors or omissions in future editions of this book.

# Contents

| | |
|---|---|
| *Citation Information* | vii |
| *Notes on Contributors* | ix |

Preface: Affordable Care Act: A Comprehensive and
Integrated Approach to Health Care     1
*Ford Kuramoto and Francis Yuen*

1. Full Immersion in the Mainstream: How Years of Promise for
   Mental Health and Substance Use Disorders Came to Fruition
   with the ACA     4
   *William Emmet, Oscar Morgan and Judy Stange*

2. Lessons Learned from a Maryland Citizen's Advocacy Group's
   Experience in Impacting Health Reform: The Seven C's of Effective
   Citizen Advocacy     21
   *Adrienne Ellis and Linda Raines*

3. Behavioral Health Parity and the Affordable Care Act     31
   *Richard Frank, Kirsten Beronio and Sherry Glied*

4. Affordable Care Act and Integrated Care     44
   *Ford Kuramoto*

5. The Affordable Care Act: Overview and Implications for County and
   City Behavioral Health and Intellectual/Developmental Disability
   Programs     87
   *Ron Manderscheid*

6. State *Olmstead* Litigation and the ACA     97
   *Terence Ng, Charlene Harrington and Alice Wong*

7. The Affordable Care Act for Behavioral Health Consumers and
   Families     110
   *Ted Johnson, David Sanders and Judy Stange*

8. Women's Health and Behavioral Health Issues in Health Care Reform     122
   *Jean Lau Chin, Barbara Yee and Martha Banks*

## CONTENTS

9. The Impact of the Affordable Care Act on the Health and Behavioral
   Health of Racial and Ethnic Minority Communities  139
   *Oscar Morgan, Ford Kuramoto, William Emmet, Judy Stange and
   Eric Nobunaga*

10. Overview of the Affordable Care Act's Impact on Military and
    Veteran Mental Health Services: Nine Implications for Significant
    Improvements in Care  162
    *Charles Figley and Mark Russell*

    *Index*  197

# Citation Information

The chapters in this book were originally published in the *Journal of Social Work in Disability & Rehabilitation*, volume 13, issues 1–2 (January–June 2014). When citing this material, please use the original page numbering for each article, as follows:

**Preface**

*The Affordable Care Act: A Comprehensive and Integrated Approach to Health Care*
Ford Kuramoto and Francis Yuen
*Journal of Social Work in Disability & Rehabilitation*, volume 13, issues 1–2 (January–June 2014) pp. 1–3

**Chapter 1**

*Full Immersion in the Mainstream: How Years of Promise for Mental Health and Substance Use Disorders Came to Fruition with the Affordable Care Act*
William Emmet, Oscar Morgan, and Judy L. Stange
*Journal of Social Work in Disability & Rehabilitation*, volume 13, issues 1–2 (January–June 2014) pp. 4–20

**Chapter 2**

*Lessons Learned from a Maryland Citizen Advocacy Group's Experience in Impacting Health Reform: The Seven Cs of Effective Citizen Advocacy*
Linda Raines and Adrienne Ellis
*Journal of Social Work in Disability & Rehabilitation*, volume 13, issues 1–2 (January–June 2014) pp. 21–30

**Chapter 3**

*Behavioral Health Parity and the Affordable Care Act*
Richard G. Frank, Kirsten Beronio, and Sherry A. Glied
*Journal of Social Work in Disability & Rehabilitation*, volume 13, issues 1–2 (January–June 2014) pp. 31–43

# CITATION INFORMATION

**Chapter 4**
*The Affordable Care Act and Integrated Care*
Ford Kuramoto
*Journal of Social Work in Disability & Rehabilitation*, volume 13, issues 1–2
(January–June 2014) pp. 44–86

**Chapter 5**
*The Affordable Care Act: Overview and Implications for County and City*
*Behavioral Health and Intellectual/Developmental Disability Programs*
Ron Manderscheid
*Journal of Social Work in Disability & Rehabilitation*, volume 13, issues 1–2
(January–June 2014) pp. 87–96

**Chapter 6**
*State* Olmstead *Litigation and the Affordable Care Act*
Terence Ng, Alice Wong, and Charlene Harrington
*Journal of Social Work in Disability & Rehabilitation*, volume 13, issues 1–2
(January–June 2014) pp. 97–109

**Chapter 7**
*The Affordable Care Act for Behavioral Health Consumers and Families*
Ted J. Johnson, David H. Sanders, and Judy L. Stange
*Journal of Social Work in Disability & Rehabilitation*, volume 13, issues 1–2
(January–June 2014) pp. 110–121

**Chapter 8**
*Women's Health and Behavioral Health Issues in Health Care Reform*
Jean Lau Chin, Barbara W. K. Yee, and Martha E. Banks
*Journal of Social Work in Disability & Rehabilitation*, volume 13, issues 1–2
(January–June 2014) pp. 122–138

**Chapter 9**
*The Impact of the Affordable Care Act on Behavioral Health Care for Individuals*
*From Racial and Ethnic Communities*
Oscar Morgan, Ford Kuramoto, William Emmet, Judy L. Stange, and Eric Nobunaga
*Journal of Social Work in Disability & Rehabilitation*, volume 13, issues 1–2
(January–June 2014) pp. 139–161

**Chapter 10**
*Overview of the Affordable Care Act's Impact on Military and Veteran Mental*
*Health Services: Nine Implications for Significant Improvements in Care*
Mark C. Russell and Charles R. Figley
*Journal of Social Work in Disability & Rehabilitation*, volume 13, issues 1–2
(January–June 2014) pp. 162–196

Please direct any queries you may have about the citations to
clsuk.permissions@cengage.com

# Notes on Contributors

**Martha E. Banks** is a research neuropsychologist at ABackans DCP, Inc., in Akron, Ohio, USA, and a former professor at The College of Wooster, Ohio, USA, and Kent State University, Ohio, USA. She is the co-author of the *Ackerman–Banks Neuropsychological Rehabilitation Battery and the Post-Assault Traumatic Brain Injury Interview & Checklist*. She co-edited *Women With Visible and Invisible Disabilities: Multiple Intersections, Multiple Issues, Multiple Therapies* (Routledge, 2003) and the three-volume book set *Disabilities: Insights from Across Fields and Around the World* (2009).

**Kristen Beronio** currently serves as Director of the Behavioral Health and Intellectual Disabilities Policy Division within the Office of the Assistant Secretary for Planning and Evaluation at the U.S. Department of Health and Human Services. Previously, she was Vice President for Public Policy and Advocacy for Mental Health America, a national non-profit organization focused on improving services and supports for individuals with mental health conditions.

**Jean Lau Chin** is a Professor at Adelphi University, New York, USA. She has held senior management positions as Dean at Alliant International University, Alhambra, California, USA, and at Adelphi University, and as Executive Director of South Cove Community Health Centre, Boston, USA, and the Thom Mental Health Clinic. As past President of the Society for the Psychology of Women, and of the Society for the Psychological Study of Ethnic Minority Issues, her presidential initiatives on leadership promoted the integration of diversity into our models of leadership and helped to advance leadership training for women and ethnic minorities.

**Adrienne Ellis** is the Director of the Maryland Parity Project, an initiative of the Mental Health Association of Maryland. In addition to outreach and education, the Maryland Parity Project staff assists providers and consumers in navigating the often complicated insurance appeals process. Before joining the Maryland Parity Project, she was the Research Director at an Annapolis-based government affairs firm. She has worked with Maryland state legislators in both health care and higher education arenas as a member of the government affairs team of the University of Maryland, Baltimore, USA.

**William Emmet** has been a mental health advocate for more than 20 years and served as Director of the Campaign for Mental Health Reform from 2006 through

2009. He also worked at the state and national levels of the National Alliance on Mental Illness. He became involved in advocacy as he supported his brother in his struggles with co-occurring mental health and substance use disorders. He also served as Project Director for Policy Analysis and Technical Assistance at the National Association of State Mental Health Program Directors, working with partners in the mental health community to provide technical assistance in policy formulation.

**Charles R. Figley** is the Distinguished Chair in Disaster Mental Health and Director of the Traumatology Institute at Tulane University, New Orleans, USA, where he is also Professor and Associate Dean in the School of Social Work. His recent books include *Encyclopedia of Trauma* (2012), the second edition of *Helping Traumatized Families* (2012), *Practitioner's Guide to Treating Traumatic Stress Injuries in Military Personnel: An EMDR Practitioner's Guide* (2013), and *First Do No Self-Harm: Understanding and Promoting Physician Stress Resilience* (2013).

**Richard G. Frank** is the Margaret T. Morris Professor of Health Economics in the Department of Health Care Policy at Harvard Medical School, Boston, USA. He is also a Research Associate with the National Bureau of Economic Research. He is engaged in research in three general areas: the economics of mental health care; the economics of the pharmaceutical industry; and the organization and financing of physician group practices. He serves on the Biobehavioral Sciences Board of the Institute of Medicine, and advises several state mental health and substance abuse agencies on issues related to managed care and financing.

**Sherry A. Glied** became Dean of the NYU Wagner School of Public Service, New York City, USA, in August 2013. She served as Assistant Secretary for Planning and Evaluation at the U.S. Department of Health and Human Services under President Obama. She was on the faculty of the Department of Health Policy and Management at Columbia University's Mailman School of Public Health. Earlier, she was a senior economist for health care and labour market policy on the President's Council of Economic Advisers under Presidents Bush and Clinton. Her most recent book, *Better But Not Well: Mental Health Policy in the U.S. Since 1950*, was published in 2006.

**Charlene Harrington** has been a professor of sociology and nursing at the University of California, San Francisco, USA, since 1980, where she has specialized in long-term care policy and research. She was elected to the Institute of Medicine (IOM) in 1996, and served on various IOM committees. In 2002, she and a team of researchers designed a model California long-term care consumer information system website funded by the California Health Care Foundation, and she continues to maintain and expand the site. In 2003, she became the principal investigator of a 5-year, $4.5 million national Center for Personal Assistance Services funded by the National Institute on Disability and Rehabilitation Research, which was refunded for 2008 through 2013.

**Ted. J. Johnson** has served since 2000 as Adjunct Faculty at the Kanawha Valley Community and Technical College, West Virginia, USA, instructing in the program for Community Behavioral Health Technology. He retired in 2002 as the Assistant Director of the West Virginia Office of Behavioral Health Services, having served

NOTES ON CONTRIBUTORS

30 years in community behavioral health services at the local and state levels. He is the Chair of the Board of Directors of the National Association of Mental Health Planning and Advisory Councils and has served as reviewer, panel chair, and review writer for the Community Mental Health Services Block Grant administered by the Substance Abuse and Mental Health Services Administration.

**Ford Kuramoto** has 30 years of experience in substance abuse and mental health services. He was on the staff of the National Institute of Mental Health in Rockville, Maryland, USA; on the faculty of the School of Medicine at UCLA, Los Angeles, USA; and the Graduate Program in Addiction Studies at Nova Southeastern University, Fort Lauderdale, Florida, USA. He served on the Behavior Change Expert Panel for the White House Office of National Drug Control Policy Media Campaign, and the Substance Abuse and Mental Health Services Administration National Advisory Council. He is also the President of Magna Systems, Inc.

**Ron Manderscheid** serves as the Executive Director of the National Association of County Behavioral Health and Developmental Disability Directors. Concurrently, he is Adjunct Professor in the Department of Mental Health, Bloomberg School of Public Health, Johns Hopkins University, Baltimore, USA, and Past President of ACMHA, The College for Behavioral Health Leadership. He serves on the boards of the Employee Assistance Research Foundation, the Danya Institute, the FrameWorks Institute, the Council on Quality and Leadership, the International Credentialing and Reciprocity Consortium, and the National Research Institute. He also serves as the Co-Chair of the Coalition for Whole Health. Throughout his career, he has emphasized and promoted peer and family concerns.

**Oscar Morgan** has more than 30 years of experience in the behavioral health field. He was the Project Director for the consultation to the Colorado health and behavioral health agencies, and was the Project Director for the Centre for Mental Health Services–funded Mental Health State Planning and Advisory Councils Project. He also worked on a Substance Abuse and Mental Health Services Administration Administrator's project regarding the behavioral health aspects of the Affordable Care Act. As former Commissioner of Mental Hygiene in Maryland, Mr. Morgan oversaw a large mental health program with 3,600 service providers, 4,000 employees, and a $770 million budget.

**Terence Ng** is an Assistant Adjunct Professor and the director overseeing home and community-based services research at the Centre for Personal Assistance Services at the University of California, San Francisco, USA, which is funded by the National Institute for Disability and Rehabilitation Research. He also directs a study of home and community-based services funded by the Kaiser Commission on Medicaid and the Uninsured. In his roles, Mr. Ng overseas the collection of Medicaid long-term support and services (LTSS) data, Olmstead lawsuit details, as well as Olmstead plans. He leads the Centre's research into LTSS within the Affordable Care Act as well as the transition into managed LTSS.

**Eric Nobunaga** has over 30 years of management and administrative experience in both the business and non-profit sectors. He has provided support to many projects including developing research, producing materials and communicating with large groups of project participants, coordinating schedules, and planning events. He has conducted many literature reviews and archival research in mental health, substance abuse and the social determinants of health. Additionally, he has studied, aggregated and analyzed a wide variety of demographic data for racial and ethnic minorities in relation to health disparities.

**Linda Raines** has led, since 1992, the Maryland Mental Health Coalition's fight to advance consumer-focused policy reform. Successful initiatives of the association include enactment of Maryland's mental health parity law, criminal justice reform legislation, and enhanced budget appropriations for mental health services. Under her leadership, the Association has significantly expanded its education and outreach programs, playing a lead role in the implementation of Mental Health First Aid in the United States, in partnership with the Maryland Department of Health and Mental Hygiene, and the National Council for Community Behavioral Health and the Missouri Department of Mental Health; and launching Maryland's first Older Adult Mental Health Web site in partnership with the Johns Hopkins Geriatric Education Center.

**Mark C. Russell** is dual-Board certified in clinical psychology and clinical child and adolescent psychology and was a postdoctoral Fellow at Harvard Medical School, Boston, USA. In collaboration with the Department of Veteran's Affairs (DVA), he organized and conducted seven joint DoD/DVA Eye Movement Desensitization and Reprocessing trainings that led to the training of more than 320 military mental health clinicians, including a 2011 training of the U.S. Army's 113th Combat Stress Control Unit, prior to deploying to Afghanistan. He is the co-author of *Treating Traumatic Stress Injuries in Military Personnel* (Routledge, 2013), and currently chairs the PsyD program at Antioch University, Seattle, USA. He is the establishing Director of the Institute of War Stress Injuries, Recovery, and Social Justice.

**David H. Sanders** has 20 years in the behavioral health care field. He has spent the last 13 years working in the non-profit arena doing systemic community and public policy advocacy at the state and local levels. He is a person in recovery from mental health and substance abuse issues, and enjoys sharing his story of recovery with others. He is an accomplished trainer and has presented nationally on public policy advocacy, psychiatric advance directives, and supported housing, protecting due process in involuntary treatment procedures. Mr. Sanders is a Board Member of the Psychiatric Rehabilitation Association, and also a Board Member of the National Coalition for Mental Health Recovery.

**Judy L. Stange** was the Co-Project Director for the Centre for Mental Health Services' Mental Health Planning and Advisory Councils (MHPAC) contract for Magna Systems, Incorporated. She addressed issues related to federal and state mental health policy and is an expert on the Mental Health Block Grant. She has more than 20 years of experience in the design of mental health and substance use disorder service systems and in behavioral health care policy. She has held positions in public and private behavioral health care settings, conducting evaluations and participating in the development of quality assurance systems.

**Alice Wong** works on various Personal Assistance Services (PAS) workforce projects for the PAS Centre. Currently, she is an author of online curricula for home care providers for Elsevier's College of Personal Assistance and Caregiving. She also conducts research on the health care needs of people with disabilities. Ms. Wong is currently the President of the San Francisco IHSS Public Authority Governing Body and a Presidential appointee to the National Council on Disability, an independent federal agency focusing on disability policy.

**Barbara W. K. Yee** is Professor and Chair of the Department of Family and Consumer Sciences at the University of Hawai'i at Mānoa, USA. Her research examines how gender, health literacy, and acculturation influence chronic disease health beliefs and lifestyle practices across three generations of Vietnamese, Asian Americans, and Pacific Islanders living in the United States. She has served on the National Institutes of Health Advisory Committee on Research on Women's Health and served on the Committee on Women.

# PREFACE

## The Affordable Care Act: A Comprehensive and Integrated Approach to Health Care

This special issue tries to capture the essence of a monumental piece of public health history and its implications for health and behavioral health care in the United States. The Patient Protection and Affordable Care Act (ACA) of 2010 is in the process of being implemented as this introduction is being written. Although the legislation is not considered perfect by many advocates, the enrollment process for ACA has begun across America. An estimated 32 million people will become eligible for health insurance. With the help of ACA, health will become a right for all Americans and the United States will finally have health reform, comprehensive health insurance, holistic integrated health and behavioral health care, along with a measure of cost control. When our team of authors started writing, we felt the enthusiasm of President Barack Obama's promise to make ACA his top domestic initiative and a hallmark of his administration and legacy. We remained undaunted, even when several states filed suit, and the U.S. Supreme Court reaffirmed the legality of most of the major provisions of ACA. Already, 3 million young adults have benefited from the provision that allows individuals to remain covered by their parents' health insurance until age 26. However, at this writing, there is opposition in Congress to the ACA legislation and some states indicate they will not fully participate in the ACA implementation. Perhaps we will have to wait to see how many eligible Americans will enroll in the Medicaid expansion provisions, the next major step in the ACA implementation. For those who enroll in the Medicaid expansion, most of whom are expected to be people of color, how satisfied will they be with the services they receive and how well will the service providers respond to the increase in demand for culturally competent, integrated, health and behavioral health services? Meanwhile, health and behavioral health care professionals, service institutions, consumers, and other stakeholders should prepare for the full implementation of ACA. Being alert to changing federal policies and being flexible and adaptive will be helpful in the coming months. We hope this special issue will assist anyone interested in seeing that ACA fulfills its promise.

This issue is organized into two sections. The first section encompasses articles that address ACA as federal policy and legislation in terms of its legislative and political history, the health reform measures, the essential health benefits, financing, advocacy efforts, and the role of integrated health care. The opening article, "Full Immersion in the Mainstream: How Years of Promise for Mental Health and Substance Use Disorders Came to Fruition With the Affordable Care Act" by William Emmet, Oscar Morgan, and Judy Stange, presents a legislative history of the Patient Protection and Affordable Care Act and the Wellstone and Domenici Mental Health and Addiction Equity Act of 2008 (MHPAEA). The article also discusses the major provisions of the ACA. It establishes the groundwork for the next four articles, which elaborate related ACA historical, policy, and program issues. The next article, "Lessons Learned From a Maryland Citizen Advocacy Group's Experience in Impacting Health Reform: The Seven Cs of Effective Citizen Advocacy" by Linda Raines and Adrienne Ellis, views the legislative history of the ACA from the perspective of citizens, consumers, and advocates, exploring how grass-roots community advocates had an impact on the formulation of federal health policy and the ACA. The article notes that the rising cost of health care was a major driving force behind the passage of the ACA. The next article by Richard G. Frank, Kirsten Beronio, and Sherry A. Glied, "Behavioral Health Parity and the Affordable Care Act," focuses on financing issues and the provisions of the ACA regarding behavioral health services and parity. "The Affordable Care Act and Integrated Care" by Ford Kuramoto provides an overview of the origins of the integrated care model in primary health care as well as behavioral health services, which the ACA ultimately merged together in its provisions. The last article in the first section is "The Affordable Care Act: Overview and Implications for County and City Behavioral Health and Intellectual/Developmental Disability Programs" by Ron Manderscheid. The article reviews the ACA with particular attention to the insurance reform aspects of the legislation and the implications for people with disabilities served by local public agencies.

The second section of this special issue includes articles that address several major segments of the populations eligible for ACA and its impact on them. This section begins with the article by Terence Ng, Alice Wong, and Charlene Harrington, "State *Olmstead* Litigation and the Affordable Care Act," which examines the U.S. Supreme Court's landmark *Olmstead v. L.C.* decision in 1999 requiring states and territories to serve people with disabilities in the community and out of institutions. The article discusses the implications of the health and behavioral health service provisions of the ACA that will help improve the care to people with disabilities in the community. As a result, ACA services will help states and territories comply with the *Olmstead* decision. Consumers of behavioral health services and their families are the subject of the article, "The Affordable Care Act for Behavioral Health Consumers and Families" by Ted J. Johnson, David H. Sanders, and Judy L. Stange. The ACA emphasizes a client-centered approach wherein consumers play an important role in determining the care they receive. The article by Jean Lau Chin, Barbara W. K. Yee, and Martha E. Banks, "Women's Health and Behavioral Health Issues in Health Care Reform," focuses on the needs of women and how the ACA addresses their special concerns. The article by Oscar Morgan, Ford Kuramoto, William Emmet, Judy Stange and Eric Nobunaga, "The Impact of the Affordable Care Act on Behavioral Health Care for Individuals From Racial and Ethnic Communities," discusses racial and ethnic minority populations. The article provides demographic profiles, rates of health and behavioral health issues, rates of insured and uninsured, and data regarding health disparities and health equity for the four major racial and ethnic minority communities. The final article addresses the health and behavioral health needs of veterans and their families. "Overview of the Affordable Care Act's Impact on Military and Veteran Mental Health Services: Nine Implications for Significant Improvements in Care" by Mark C. Russell and Charles R. Figley describes the many types of military, veteran, and civilian health services available to current veterans and their families. The ACA will add to the health and behavioral health care options available to them.

These articles present an in-depth look at the Patient Protection and Affordable Care Act of 2010 from a variety of perspectives. As evidenced by these articles the ACA provides the first comprehensive and integrated approach to health care in over 50 years. The implementation of the ACA will provide much needed health care services and other resources, particularly for some of the most vulnerable and needy populations in the United States. The hope is that this special issue will help illuminate the path forward for consumers, service providers, and policymakers as ACA makes health a right.

Ford Kuramoto, *Guest Editor*
Francis Yuen, *Editor-in-Chief*

# Full Immersion in the Mainstream: How Years of Promise for Mental Health and Substance Use Disorders Came to Fruition with the Affordable Care Act

WILLIAM EMMET, OSCAR MORGAN, and JUDY L. STANGE

*Magna Systems, Inc., Largo, Maryland, USA*

*With passage of the Patient Protection and Affordable Care Act (ACA), the behavioral health community has achieved entry into the mainstream of U.S. health care. Passage of the law was the culmination of a long effort by advocates. At the same time, findings from research and practice have informed the nation's understanding that behavioral health is integral to health. The primary task before the behavioral health community now is to ensure that the advances of recent years are secured through implementation of the ACA and approaches to service delivery that emphasize integrated care.*

When President Barack Obama signed the Patient Protection and Affordable Care Act (ACA or, colloquially, Obamacare) on March 23, 2010, few but the most attentive behavioral health advocates fully appreciated its implications for those needing treatment for substance abuse or mental health disorders.[1] In fact, the ACA was both the signal achievement of the decades-long movement for improved mental health and substance abuse service availability and the gateway to an uncertain world in which the contours of access and services will likely be unclear for years to come. It is well worth reflecting on how behavioral health services came to be included in the ACA, and it is very important to understand how the legislative victory can turn to dust if implementation of the law and the practices it encourages are not handled carefully.

## SEPARATE SYSTEMS

Until passage of the ACA, the history of mental health and substance use disorder treatment in this country unfolded largely outside the broader health care system. Much has been written about why this is so, but, until very recently, the effect was that most discussion of health system reform largely overlooked these illnesses and disorders. This was true as recently as the short-lived effort to reform health care undertaken during the Clinton administration in 1993 and 1994. Although mental health was included in the early rounds of those discussions, once policymakers got serious, it was pushed off the table on the shared assumption that coverage for mental health treatments would be prohibitively expensive.

Similar reasoning had been behind the decision in 1965 to put psychiatric hospitals in a separate class, ineligible for reimbursement under the new Medicaid program. At the time, it was commonly understood that diagnoses of serious mental illness (SMI) signaled a lifetime of hospitalization. The concept of recovery, the goal of services provided today, had not yet entered the thinking of most mental health professionals and policymakers, most of whom believed that mental illness was irreversible, with treatment serving mainly to "control" symptoms that might erupt at any time.

Beginning in the 19th century, every state operated institutions that at their peak housed more than 500,000 Americans, many in deplorable conditions far removed from public consciousness. Keeping these institutions running was the business of state departments of mental health, charged with maintaining the grounds and buildings the patients occupied and with managing the substantial workforce required to look after people who had nowhere else to turn for shelter, food, or care. Under the Medicaid law, these institutions, once thought of as peaceful asylums where people with mental health problems could find peace as they grappled with their demons, were categorized as "institutions for mental diseases" (IMDs) that could not receive funds provided for services to the poor or people living with other medical conditions. Only with the Community Mental Health Act, signed into law by President Kennedy in 1963, did public policy begin to reflect the slow changes in public understanding of mental illnesses and support for community-based services.

Parallel to the physical segregation experienced by so many with mental illnesses was the denial of medical care to those receiving any kind of mental health diagnosis. In part, this was a result of the general assumption that once a mental disorder had been diagnosed, a person's life was as good as over. Indeed, many family members were told by doctors or other mental health professionals that they should behave as if their mentally ill son, daughter, sibling, or spouse were dead. That being the case, the only care they needed would be custodial; with no hope for recovery, medical interventions were not seen as necessary.

Not all family members took this awful advice, of course, but most ran up against a very practical reality, which was the inability to find health insurance that would cover someone with a mental health diagnosis. For those seeking insurance, mental health problems constituted a preexisting condition that simply made a person ineligible for any coverage. Some were fortunate enough to become insured before mental illness reared its head, only to find they would reach arbitrarily set limits in the number of hospital days or outpatient visits covered or the amount of money that could be paid out for such services. Once those limits were reached, insurance was no longer obtainable. Many families spent themselves into poverty by paying for uncovered services. In time, however, most found they had to settle for state services or none at all due to the unyielding policies imposed by insurers.

Even the federal government found the costs of covering mental health treatment, such as it was, to be prohibitive, as illustrated by the "IMD exclusion" from Medicaid reimbursement.[2] The Medicare program, too, has long placed limits on the psychiatric services it pays for, a problem that has not yet been fully addressed, even to this day.[3] States, therefore, remained largely responsible for the system of last resort for people with mental health conditions. Only with significant changes in approach did states find a way to share this burden with federal and, sometimes, local payors.

As the deinstitutionalization movement begun in the 1960s gained steam through the 1980s, people with mental health diagnoses and their families found traction as advocates. They focused on the state mental health systems and the federal agencies charged with regulating them, systems that made life in the community their chief goal. They became deeply embroiled in trying to make the separate systems created to provide community-based services for people with mental illnesses responsive to their needs, even as the pain and stigma they experienced resulted in large measure from the existence of those separate systems.

## PARITY

One line of advocacy that began in the late 1980s and gained traction in the early 1990s was focused on erasing a major inequity perpetuating the separate systems: the limitations placed by insurance policies on the coverage they provided for mental illnesses. For many family members and their relatives with mental health diagnoses, problems with private insurance seemed irrelevant. Having exhausted their coverage early in the course of their illness, the majority of adults with SMIs—those who would at one time have been hospitalized in state institutions—were more concerned with maintaining and improving the benefits offered by public systems. Yet, some of these advocates saw that in the long run insurance "parity" could help bring people with mental illnesses back into the health care mainstream. More important, from an advocacy perspective, they understood that a campaign for parity could present a perfect opportunity to put the inequities associated with mental illness—stigma, inadequate services, insufficient research, unfair insurance rules, and a host of other discriminatory practices—on public display. An effective campaign to achieve insurance parity could drive a much broader policy discussion focused on placing mental health in the social and health care mainstream.

The ensuing campaign spearheaded by advocacy organizations such as NAMI and what was then known as the National Mental Health Association,[4] in close alliance with the American Psychiatric Association and other professional trade groups, unfolded first on the state level and within a few years gained momentum as a federal issue. Significantly, the idea that mental illnesses should be treated by insurance companies "like any other condition" found adherents among state and federal legislators with family members who had experienced the very discrimination parity legislation was meant to address. Most prominently, Senators Paul Wellstone (D-MN) and Pete Domenici (R-NM) stepped onto the floor of the U.S. Senate to reveal that mental illness affected close relatives. By 1996, enough support had been gathered for Congress to send President Clinton a limited Mental Health Parity Act, which he readily signed.

For advocates, passage of the Mental Health Parity Act of 1996 was empowering, encouraging, and a spur to further action. Because the law was so limited,[5] advocates could hardly declare the battle won, but they had tasted success and understood that parity was an issue that resonated with policymakers across the partisan divide. Only half the battle was taking place at the federal level, where the typical "self-insured" large employer plans are regulated under authority of the Employee Retirement Income Security Act of 1974 (ERISA).[6] Most insurance plans applying to smaller employers and individual subscribers are regulated by states. Starting in 1994 with New Hampshire, Rhode Island, and Maryland, an increasing number of state legislatures passed laws bringing some degree of parity to coverage of mental health disorders.[7] For policymakers in statehouses and the U.S. Capitol, the words *mental health parity*—and the concepts behind them— were becoming very familiar.

## CLINTON HEALTH REFORM

The march toward parity gained momentum late in President Clinton's first term. It was a mere blip on the screen, however, when compared with the major health reform effort mounted by the Clinton administration in 1993 and 1994, its first years in office. Behind closed doors, a huge task force led by then–First Lady Hillary Clinton and policy guru Ira Magaziner pieced together a mammoth restructuring of the nation's health care payment and delivery systems. Employing a strategy whose failure would heavily influence President Obama's approach 16 years later, the idea was to present Congress with a fully drafted bill. At the start of the process, even before Clinton's inauguration, indications were that mental health would be woven into the new plan as part of a comprehensive health reform effort. Strong voices on the task force and within the administration kept mental health on the table during the early phases of the discussions. However, as concerns mounted about the rising costs of the plan, it became clear that its designers were prepared to leave mental health by the side as health care was reformed. In the end, of course, the entire Clinton health reform effort could not navigate the treacherous political waters onto which it had sailed; it sank without ever coming to a vote in Congress.

Clinton's health reform failure left behind many lessons for anyone interested in the nexus of policy and politics. For mental health advocates, one lesson was that no matter what assurances they might have been given, mental health was seen as an expendable component of overall health care when the going got rough. Many vowed that if the opportunity ever arose again, they would be better prepared to make the case that mental health was integral to health.

## SPOTLIGHT ON MENTAL HEALTH

Although the first-term health reform effort failed, the Clinton administration in 1999 provided two significant platforms on which advocates and health policy experts could subsequently make their case. One, the White House Conference on Mental Health, allowed a media spotlight to be shone on the issue, and the other, a report of the U.S. Surgeon General on mental health, provided a wealth of scientific information that to this day informs policymakers on the causes, epidemiology, and treatments of mental health disorders.

On a sweltering day in June 1999, the White House Conference brought together several hundred legislators, administration officials, scientists, state administrators, doctors, nurses, and other professionals with advocates, family members, and people with the lived experience of mental illness, all to discuss promising approaches to providing appropriate supports to those needing them. The strongest message, however, was conveyed by the appearance of President and Mrs. Clinton together on a stage with Vice President and Mrs. Gore spending several hours discussing mental health as a national policy issue. Mental health had demonstrably captured the attention of the nation's highest officials.

*Mental Health: A Report of the Surgeon General* (U.S. Department of Health and Human Services, 1999) is a hefty volume that remains one of the foundational documents for present-day advocates. Steeped in science, it provides a clear picture of the toll mental disorders take on the lives of Americans, while pointing to the best approaches to prevention, wellness, and recovery from SMI. It very clearly examines mental health in a public health context, showing that "there is no health without mental health." The report also zeroes in on the destructive role played by stigma in preventing the public from understanding mental health, keeping people who need it away from treatment, and blinding policymakers to the role they should play in providing the funds for necessary preventive and treatment services.

The Surgeon General's report elevated the mental health policy discussion to a new level, leading to a much more integrative view of mental health and paving the way for several later reports from different bodies, most notably the Institute of Medicine, which has now issued reports, among others, on improving the quality of care for people with mental health and substance use disorders (National Research Council, 2006); on prevention of mental, emotional, and behavioral disorders among young people (National Research Council, 2009); and on the mental health and substance use workforce for older adults (National Research Council, 2012).

## PRESIDENT BUSH'S NEW FREEDOM COMMISSION

In terms of policy and public perception, the most important sequel to the 1999 White House Conference and the Surgeon General's Report might well have been the creation of the President's New Freedom Commission on Mental Health by George W. Bush in 2002 and release of the report it produced in 2003 (New Freedom Commission on Mental Health, 2003). In the eyes of many advocates, the mere existence of the Commission, created as it was by a Republican president, demonstrated the nonpartisan nature of mental health policy. The report, which reflected countless hours of testimony and meetings, was packaged for easier consumption than the Surgeon General's report (U.S. Department of Health and Human Services, 1999) had been. It was organized around six goals; a decade later, they retain their immediacy for national mental health policy, and, most significantly, they align closely with goals set forth 7 years later in the Affordable Care Act.[8]

Both the Surgeon General's report (U.S. Department of Health and Human Services, 1999) and the New Freedom Commission on Mental Health (2003) report recognized the host of broader public policy issues clearly connected to mental health. They documented numerous failures in mental health policy. The high-level attention given by these reports to complex social problems connected with mental health gave support to efforts underway to develop collaborative responses to them.

Rising homelessness, for instance, had long been seen as a consequence of the failure to fully fund community mental health services or hold them accountable for serving the deinstitutionalized population. Although some studies debunked the easy notion that every homeless person on a given city street should be hospitalized—or would have been in an earlier time—let alone the casual belief that every homeless person had a mental illness, the nagging truth was that many on the streets remained untouched by a system most in the public supposed was there to serve them. But it wasn't just the mental health service system that had let homeless people down. The cost of housing was rising beyond the means of a growing number of people in many cities and towns, and policies followed by housing agencies ensured that many people with mental illnesses would not be offered safe and affordable places to live.

Another example of a social quandary arising from inadequately addressed mental health issues can be found at the intersection of the criminal justice and mental health systems. Here, there was a history of finger pointing and a sense that the two cultures—criminal justice and mental health—could not find common ground. Mental health advocates, providers, family members, and clients cited endless instances of brutality committed by law enforcement officers, jailers, and prison authorities. At the same time, the criminal justice community was frustrated with a mental health community that allowed people with untreated mental illness to wander the streets and cause public nuisances that kept officers from their broader public safety role. All were fed up with the overcrowded jails and the clogged courtrooms resulting from the repeated arrests and detention of so many people with mental illnesses.

These rounds of recrimination were frustrating to public officials and policymakers, some of whom came to realize that solutions to these accumulating problems would require cooperation and collaboration across the boundaries each system had erected. Collaborative projects emerged in scattered communities, and private foundations and the federal government sought partners among national organizations able to identify effective approaches and help more communities to replicate them. There was a clear recognition that lives were being wasted as a result of ineffective policies, but action on these issues was also motivated by the unavoidable fact that they represented a very poor use of the public dollar. The "Housing First" model, for example, was seen as a way to cut through red tape that had prevented many people disabled by mental illness, substance abuse, or other conditions from moving into stable homes.[9] It gained support when it was shown that many formerly homeless people made their way to stable housing through this approach, which also had the advantage of being far less costly than the endless cycle of failed treatment, hospitalization, or frequent visits to jail (Larimer et al., 2009).

Similarly, the Council of State Governments' Criminal Justice/Mental Health Consensus Project highlighted ways in which, working across boundaries, the criminal justice and mental health systems could reduce deadly confrontations between police and mentally ill persons, help clear court calendars clogged by cases complicated by mental health issues, and forge connections that would cut recidivism rates for people with mental illnesses released from jails and prisons.[10] Looked at through the eyes of elected and appointed officials, these steps reduced budget pressures and made better use of public funds; they were good policy and good politics.

Efforts to address such thorny policy issues affected clinical perceptions as well. Homeless people, for example, are rarely if ever found to suffer from mental illness alone. Many might also chronically abuse substances, be HIV-positive, or have significant pulmonary issues. As clinicians began to report more regularly on cooccurring diagnoses, policy discussions, in turn, became more encompassing. In the early 2000s, therefore, the traditional concept of SMI became much more layered. Yes, clinicians found an underlying mental illness might have led someone into poverty and homelessness; however, the trauma, both emotional and physical, that resulted from these circumstances often contributed its own disabling effects to that person's overall clinical picture.

More clinicians and mental health policy experts became aware of the inescapable fact that a high percentage of people in the mental health system had experienced some form of trauma, often repeated, during their lives. Further investigation showed this to be true of many men and women identified as having mental health disorders in the criminal justice system, as well. This understanding has led to a reconsideration of long-used clinical practices. The effort to reduce the use of seclusion and restraints spread from psychiatric hospitals even into some parts of state and county correctional systems. At a minimum, many clinicians came to recognize the value in understanding a person's "trauma history" in assessing his or her behavior and developing therapeutic interventions.

Beginning in the late 1990s, the Adverse Childhood Experiences (ACE) Study and a variety of follow-up efforts provided support for understanding the consequences of trauma (Felitti et al., 1998). The ACE study certainly detailed what might be called the psychological consequences of trauma, but the real breakthrough it facilitated was in understanding that a large number of somatic conditions could also be traced back to trauma in childhood. By the early 2000s, the concept that trauma might underlie many mental and somatic conditions was gaining followers and scientific credence.

The connection between trauma and mental health disorders was made relentlessly clear during the first decade of the 21st century by the growing recognition that men and women in the armed forces were experiencing posttraumatic stress disorder (PTSD) and substance abuse problems at previously unrecorded rates, with a record number taking their own lives. With many soldiers deployed to Iraq and Afghanistan multiple times and the all-volunteer military stretched thin, the problem of trauma-related behavioral health disorders rose dramatically in the public's consciousness.

Services for these disorders appeared to be inadequate. Active-duty soldiers, recognizing that any intimation of behavioral health problems would blot their records and end their prospects for advancement and promotion, mostly stayed away from clinics until their problems were unavoidable and severe. At the same time, veterans attempting to use the services of the Veterans Health Administration encountered many roadblocks from a bureaucracy seemingly intent on holding down disability payouts and medical benefits.

It has become axiomatic that every war brings unanticipated changes to civilian society. For post-9/11 combat, one area of significant spillover has come in our nation's understanding of certain mental disorders. With so many of those deployed coming from the National Guard and Reserves, civilian behavioral health service providers found themselves faced with clinical presentations for which they were initially unprepared. Necessity has brought innovation in many practices, including, most notably, a strong reliance on peer support for many struggling with their combat-related disorders in military and veteran health care settings, as well as in a civilian service array that has become more welcoming to those with military backgrounds.

Advancing awareness of behavioral health consequences of the particular types of asymmetrical combat experienced by so many of those deployed to war zones and increased recognition of the physical effects of the percussive explosions have helped to focus brain research, as well. In his post-Congressional career, Patrick Kennedy has helped to start the One Mind Campaign,[11] which is devoted to uniting the disease-specific brain research enterprise into one integrated effort that, the Campaign suggests, will benefit all afflicted with brain disorders.

A shared complaint of most soldiers and veterans who have experienced behavioral health problems is that stigma stands in the way of help-seeking and access to treatment, but it is also likely that the public's recognition of the disorders' prevalence among those associated with the military has led to greater acceptance of them among the nation's policy leaders.

## PREVENTABLE HEALTH PROBLEMS

In 2006, the National Association of State Mental Health Program Directors' (NASMHPD) Medical Directors Council published a study showing that people diagnosed with serious mental illnesses who received services in public mental health systems died, on average, 25 years earlier than people in the general population (NASMHPD Medical Directors Council, 2006a). Most shockingly, the study found, the health problems contributing to this dark statistic were largely preventable. For the first time, mental health policy experts and advocates were forced to examine practices within their system that allowed so many lives to end prematurely. More broadly, the study was another reminder that maintenance of a separate mental health system could be harmful to the health of the very people it was meant to serve.

One easily identifiable area in which practice could be modified to improve the overall health of people with mental health diagnoses was smoking and tobacco use. Here, too, the NASMHPD Medical Directors produced groundbreaking work, a study of smoking policy and treatment in state-operated psychiatric facilities (NASMHPD Medical Directors Council, 2006b). Simultaneously, evidence collected by the Smoking Cessation Leadership Center at the University of California, San Francisco, showed that 44% of adults with serious mental illness are smokers, compared with about 20% for society at large.[12] As administrators came to understand the harm smoking could bring to the people under their supervision, they joined the rest of society in placing restrictions on smoking in most of the physical settings they controlled.

For many years, when members of the mental health community mentioned a "dual diagnosis," the reference was to cooccurring substance use and mental health disorders. In other words, there has long been an awareness that substance abuse and forms of mental illness frequently came in one package. It is a historical oddity, therefore, that two rigidly distinct systems developed and have been maintained to address mental health and substance use disorder diagnoses. Although the two systems remain separated in many places, as the nation moves toward a much more integrated future, here, too, there have been encouraging signs of a more comprehensive, person-centered approach.

From a policy perspective, the merger of the public substance abuse and mental health treatment systems has been underway for some time. According to the Substance Abuse and Mental Health Services Administration (SAMHSA), substance abuse services were the responsibility of the state mental health agency in 31 states in 2010, but mental health and substance abuse were located in the same umbrella agency in an additional 15 states (SAMHSA, 2011, p. 10). Many would agree, however, that these organizational arrangements do not guarantee integration in funding, provider relations, or treatment philosophy. With separate block grants still enshrined in federal statutes, and a host of regulatory barriers at the federal and state levels, it will still be some time before the systems lose their separate identities. However, significant policy developments leading up to enactment of the ACA point to the embrace of a more comprehensive behavioral health approach in coming years.

## PARITY, AT LAST

The legislative process favors development of language that is more inclusive and comprehensive, if only because this is likely to build support for a proposed bill across wider constituencies. In the case of the mental health parity legislation proposed to extend and improve on the Mental Health

Parity Act of 1996, drafters bent to pressure from the addiction treatment community to include drug and alcohol abuse disorders with the mental health disorders that would be guaranteed insurance coverage. Broadening the scope of the legislation ensured support from a wider range of interest groups outside of Congress and from a larger number of legislators on both sides of the aisle on Capitol Hill. The major push for this broader approach came from the House, where Congressman Patrick Kennedy (D-RI), who had revealed his own mental health diagnosis in 2000, was joined as sponsor by Congressman Jim Ramstad (R-MN), himself in long-term recovery from alcohol abuse. Together, they won a broadening of the proposed legislation in its Senate version, as well. In so doing, they helped to build a growing army of supporters who regularly lobbied members of Congress to pass the law.

Yet, year in and year out, the bill never seemed to come up for a vote. As health reform became an issue in the 2008 election, some became worried that parity would be left behind as policymakers directed their attention to larger coverage and payment issues. Indeed, as the 110th Congress wound down and prepared for its departure before the November 2008 elections, it appeared that time had once again run out for parity legislation. It was a tremendous surprise, therefore, when the bill became the beneficiary of parliamentary maneuvering necessary to secure passage of the Troubled Asset Relief Program (TARP), a high priority for members of both parties as the nation's financial crisis was coming to a head. After years of languishing in committee, the Mental Health Parity and Addiction Equity Act (MHPAEA) of 2008, included in TARP, was passed into law and signed by President George W. Bush in one momentous day, October 3, 2008. Behavioral health advocates celebrated not just the abrupt enactment of the law, but the fact that it constituted a backstop to prevent slippage should work begin in earnest on health reform after the election.

Perhaps because the years-long struggle for parity had reached its conclusion with a dizzying final flourish, few reflected on two significant by-products of the protracted effort. One was the alliance, still somewhat uneasy, that had been formed between advocates for the addictions and mental health communities. A second, subtler bonus was the heightened understanding of mental health issues now shared by most Congressional offices. Year in and year out since at least 1996, scientists and doctors, advocates, family members, and people living with mental health diagnoses had made regular visits to Capitol Hill, repeating a consistent message: "Mental illnesses are real. Treatment works." The kicker, of course, was that without insurance coverage, many had no access to effective treatments.

## "OBAMACARE" COMES INTO FOCUS

Barack Obama's victory in the 2008 presidential election and the attainment of Democratic majorities in both the House and Senate came just a month after the passage of MHPAEA and paved the way for development of health reform legislation. Policy experts and behavioral health advocates watched closely, mindful of their issues' early removal from the table in 1993 and 1994. As the presidential campaign unfolded, behavioral health advocates worked together to develop a common policy platform and share it with advisors for the two candidates. Meetings with these advisors were arranged, and behavioral health was clearly considered part of the overall health care puzzle that policymakers seemed poised to address.

With the election over, the pace of activity picked up, and representatives of the behavioral health community were invited to present testimony before the Senate Health, Education, Labor, and Pensions (HELP) Committee, to work with the other committees of jurisdiction on both sides of the Hill, and to participate in the White House Health Reform Summit that was convened to put many of the issues on the table.[13] As debate over what eventually became the ACA dragged on over the next year, behavioral health advocates found a level of receptivity they had not expected for full inclusion of mental health and substance abuse in the bill. Although the partisan wrangling over the bill kept its fate in doubt until its very passage in March 2010, behavioral health advocates could see that their many years of effort, particularly on parity, had paid off in acceptance of mental health and addiction disorders as "conditions like any others," at least in the closely split verdict of the U.S. Congress.

The ACA included treatment for substance abuse and mental health conditions among the "essential health benefits" for which the health insurance exchanges created by the law must provide coverage. Furthermore, the ACA explicitly built on the foundation laid by MHPAEA to guarantee true parity, not the limited benefits that, it is easy to forget, were deemed progress by legislators a mere decade and a half earlier.

The ACA, for all its ambitions and flaws, incorporated to one degree or another many of the policy priorities identified by the mental health and addictions communities over the preceding 15 years. It is the first goal of the President's New Freedom Commission on Mental Health (2003) on which we should focus, however, because it sets the stage for implementation of the others and, more important, for how we should regard the law *in toto*. That first goal, "Americans understand that mental health is integral to health," actually plays out in the integrated approach the ACA encourages. The mental health needs of many Americans can be met by the primary care system and the referrals made from it to the specialty system, just as is the case for any health condition.


## MOVING TOWARD 2014

The May 19, 2012 ruling of the U.S. Supreme Court and the November 2012 reelection of Barack Obama sustained the ACA and removed the obstacles remaining in the way of implementation of the law itself and the broader move toward achievement of the "triple aim" (Berwick, Nolan, & Whittington, 2008)—better care, better health, and lower cost—regarded by former acting CMS Director Donald Berwick as central to the nation's health reform efforts. Even though states could still exercise options determining the organization of their health insurance exchanges (state-run, federally run, or run by a state–federal partnership) and whether they would accept the generous federal match in return for expanding access to services reimbursed by Medicaid, it was clear the law would not be turned back, as its opponents had fervently hoped. The regulatory apparatus at the federal Department of Health and Human Services went into overdrive once the law was upheld, and guidance on many provisions flowed to the states.

The ACA gives states substantial responsibility for creating the infrastructure needed to support reform. Therefore, the states' ability to comprehend and prepare for their role in the law's implementation is key to the entire effort's success. Early in the legislative process, lawmakers made the decision to expand coverage by having states, not the federal government, operate the exchanges and expand their existing Medicaid programs. This was seen in part as a way to avoid the charge that the new law would be a massive expansion of federal bureaucracy; it was also understood that this approach would likely be less disruptive to established insurance markets and more responsive to system peculiarities in each state. Over a year and a half after the ACA became law, the Department of Health and Human Services (HHS) issued a rule giving states responsibility for selection of the "benchmark" plans on which the benefits offered through each state's exchange would be modeled (*Essential Health Benefits Bulletin,* 2011). One effect of these decisions, however, might be perpetuation of the uneven access to services characteristic of our current system.

The Supreme Court ruling on the ACA gave states great leeway in implementing the law's Medicaid expansion provision.[14] Despite the enticement of a 100% federal contribution to reimbursement for services for the expanded Medicaid population in those states choosing the path made voluntary by the ruling, some states made the decision not to broaden Medicaid in the first year the program is available. However, the Medicaid expansion decision played out surprisingly in other states, where determined advocacy efforts succeeded in convincing even governors and legislators with ideologically hardened positions to accept the federal match by expanding coverage.

The cumulative effect of these provisions and regulations is that states have been and will continue to be presented with ongoing decisions about coverage and benefits under the ACA, many of them disproportionately affecting people with mental health or substance use conditions. Indeed, the decisions made in states in the months before the major ACA provisions become effective, and in the first year or so in which the mechanisms established by the law are operational, will go far in determining whether it fulfills its promise. The actions taken by state officials will in many ways be definitive, but everyone with a stake in the health care delivery system will have an opportunity to help shape the new environment. For this reason, health reform is a societal challenge; and for this reason, as well, implementation is likely to be inconsistent for some time.

A number of questions applying directly to behavioral health care remain to be answered as implementation moves forward. The ability of behavioral health providers to forge relationships in accountable care organizations (ACOs)—and all that means for practice and payment—is one area waiting for answers. If they fail to do so, can they survive? Or, will some other business model emerge to meet as yet unidentified needs?

At the same time, we have to ask whether individuals will be motivated to seek and receive mental health and substance use treatment in integrated or primary care settings. Will the safety net services relied on by people with serious, disabling conditions survive? Is it possible their funding will be cut off under the presumption that people will find adequate services in as yet untried integrated settings? What then?

## SECURING ADVANCES

For much of the nation's history, mental health policy has been a search for the most effective means of crisis intervention. Only recently has the conversation turned toward concepts like prevention, early intervention, and integration with general health care. This willingness to look upstream at new approaches, supported by science as well as cost considerations, has begun to affect the organization of systems, payment models, and other concrete manifestations of the way care is approached. ACOs and the health home model adopted by Medicaid for a demonstration are two innovations known or understood until recently by very few. As the ACA takes hold, however, ACOs and health homes become harbingers of behavioral health's integration into the nation's overall approach to health and well-being.

Just as policymakers, advocates, and practitioners began to grow accustomed to the idea of integration, energy for a very different discussion of behavioral health erupted from the Newtown school shooting and the widespread public view that mental illness must somehow explain the actions of the young man who committed that act. It is sadly ironic that calls for more repressive policies and, for some at least, a turn back toward separation and isolation have surged just when the nation appeared to be opening avenues by which behavioral health could join the wider health care world. These simultaneous thrusts seem to manifest the findings of a recent report indicating that although Americans recognize that mental health conditions are real illnesses, they remain fearful of the people who have them (Pescosolido, Medina, Martin, & Long, 2013).

The question of how our nation should deliver mental health services has been finding shifting answers for at least 50 years. The work done over that time by advocates and policymakers—including many directly affected by mental health disorders—has helped us to see that mental health conditions and, more important, the people who have them do belong in the mainstream of our health care and social service systems. The ACA is the largest single move toward integrated care in the nation's history, and it reflects the quiet yet relentless effort of many people. Yet, as the influence of Newtown shows us, the work is by no means over. In fact, some would say the stakes are higher than ever. Incomplete or unsuccessful integration might spark a backlash characterized by a retrenchment of the "separate but unequal" policies of the past. Knowing what we know now about people with mental health diagnoses, and knowing the potential of brain science to come, such a retrenchment would be a sad and unnecessary outcome.

To cement the place of behavioral health in the new health care environment, all stakeholders will need to work in ways that are different from any familiar to them in the past. They will need to continue to expand their vision and their universe as behavioral health moves further into the mainstream. With MHPAEA and the ACA, there are now legislative tools to support this trend, and the field is brimming with enthusiasm for these changes, but there are also many conservative forces at work that could slow or impede their adoption. Supporters of change must recognize these forces and identify effective strategies for defeating them. In the end, however, as the steady march of the past 25 to 50 years demonstrates, there is no substitute for perseverance. More than any other, advocates and their allies must continue to exhibit this quality if the changes they have achieved are to endure.

## NOTES

1. The term *behavioral health* is fully embraced by few advocates or practitioners from either the mental health or substance abuse communities, but it has become the de facto comprehensive label understood to encompass the two conditions.

2. The IMD prohibition has continued to generate controversy to the present day. Whereas some credit it with forcing states to develop and fund community-based services, others see it as inherently discriminatory, leaving potential patients without access to services they need.

3. Under the Medicare Improvement Act of 2008, the Medicare program is gradually improving mental health benefits to bring them closer to the standard set by the Mental Health Parity and Addiction Equity Act (MHPAEA), which does not apply to Medicare. Generally, by 2014, Medicare patients will pay a 20% copay for mental health care. For more information, see http://www.medicare.gov/publications/pubs/pdf/10184.pdf

4. Until 2005, NAMI's full name was the National Alliance for the Mentally Ill. The name was changed to National Alliance on Mental Illness to better reflect the "person first" language espoused by the organization. The National Mental Health Association (NMHA) changed its name in 2006 to Mental Health America.

5. The Mental Health Parity Act of 1996 did not require employers to offer mental health coverage, but did require mental health coverage, if offered, to be on a par with coverage for other conditions, as defined by the law. It applied only to employers of more than 50 employees. It did not apply to substance use or chemical dependency. It did not apply to Medicare or Medicaid, and it put no restrictions on managed care practices affecting mental health services.

THE AFFORDABLE CARE ACT AND INTEGRATED BEHAVIORAL HEALTH CARE

6. For more information on ERISA, access http://www.dol.gov/compliance/laws/comp-erisa.htm

7. Texas implemented parity for state employees in 1991, providing a model of sorts for the states that brought reforms in the broader marketplace a few years later.

8. The goals of the President's New Freedom Commission are as follows:

Goal 1: Americans understand that mental health is essential to overall health.

Goal 2: Mental health care is consumer and family driven.

Goal 3: Disparities in mental health services are eliminated.

Goal 4: Early mental health screening, assessment, and referral to services are common practice.

Goal 5: Excellent mental health care is delivered and research is accelerated.

Goal 6: Technology is used to access mental health care and information.

9. Housing First was pioneered by Pathways to Housing in 1992. To find out more about this model, see http://www.pathwaystohousing.org.

10. The Criminal Justice/Mental Health Consensus Project is an ongoing program of the Council of State Governments Justice Center. For more information on the project, see http://consensusproject.org.

11. See http://1mind4research.org/about-one-mind.

12. See http://smokingcessationleadership.ucsf.edu/MentalHealth.htm.

13. See the testimony of William Emmet before the Senate HELP Committee, January 22, 2009 at http://www.asph.org/UserFiles/Emmet%20Testimony.pdf, and a summary of the White House Forum on Health Reform, March 5, 2009, at http://www.whitehouse.gov/assets/documents/White_House_Forum_on_Health_Reform_Report.pdf

14. HHS guidance has made it clear that any state could subsequently opt to expand their Medicaid program. However, the timetable for reduction of the 100% federal match to 90% by 2019 would remain in effect.

# REFERENCES

Berwick, D. M., Nolan, T. W., & Whittington, J. (2008). The triple aim: Care, health, and cost. *Health Affairs, 27*, 759–769.

*Essential health benefits bulletin.* (2011). Baltimore, MD: Center for Consumer Information and Insurance Oversight. Retrieved from http://cciio.cms.gov/resources/files/Files2/12162011/essential_health_benefits_bulletin.pdf

Felitti, V. J., Anda, R. F., Nordenberg, D., Williamson, D. F., Spitz, A. M., Edwards, V., . . . Marks, J. S. (1998). Relationship of childhood abuse and household dysfunction to many of the leading causes of death in adults: The Adverse Childhood Experiences (ACE) study. *American Journal of Preventive Medicine, 14*, 245–258.

Larimer, M. E., Malone, D. K., Garner, M. D., Atkins, D. C., Burlingham, B., Lonczak, H. S., . . . Marlatt, G. A. (2009). Health care and public service use and costs before and after provision of housing for chronically homeless persons with severe alcohol problems. *Journal of the American Medical Association, 301*, 1349–1357. doi:10.1001/jama.2009.414

National Association of State Mental Health Program Directors Medical Directors Council. (2006a). *Morbidity and mortality in people with serious mental illness.* Retrieved from http://www.nasmhpd.org/docs/publications/MDCdocs/Mortality%20and%20Morbidity%20Final%20Report%208.18.08.pdf

National Association of State Mental Health Program Directors Medical Directors Council. (2006b). *Technical report on smoking policy and treatment in state operated psychiatric facilities.* Retrieved from http://www.nasmhpd.org/docs/

publications/MDCdocs/Oct2006%20Final%20Report%200n%20Smoking%20 Policy%20and%20Treatment%20atState%200perated%20Psychiatric%20Facilities.pdf

National Research Council. (2006). *Improving the quality of health care for mental and substance-use conditions: Quality chasm series*. Washington, DC: National Academies Press.

National Research Council. (2009). *Preventing mental, emotional, and behavioral disorders among young people: Progress and possibilities*. Washington, DC: National Academies Press.

National Research Council. (2012). *The mental health and substance use workforce for older adults: In whose hands?* Washington, DC: National Academies Press.

New Freedom Commission on Mental Health. (2003). *Achieving the promise: Transforming mental health care in America. Final report* (DHHS Pub. No. SMA-03-3832). Rockville, MD: U.S. Department of Health and Human Services.

Pescosolido, B. A., Medina, T. R., Martin, J. K., & Long, J. S. (2013). The "backbone" of stigma: Identifying the global core of public prejudice associated with mental illness. *American Journal of Public Health, 103*, 853–860. doi:10.2105/ AJPH.2012.301147

Substance Abuse and Mental Health Services Administration. (2011). *Funding and characteristics of state mental health agencies, 2010*. Rockville, MD: Author.

U.S. Department of Health and Human Services. (1999). *Mental health: A report of the Surgeon General*. Rockville, MD: U.S. Department of Health and Human Services.

# Lessons Learned from a Maryland Citizen Advocacy Group's Experience in Impacting Health Reform: The Seven Cs of Effective Citizen Advocacy

LINDA RAINES and ADRIENNE ELLIS

*Mental Health Association of Maryland, Lutherville, Maryland, USA*

*The Affordable Care Act and the Mental Health Parity and Addiction Equity Act, in conjunction with state reform efforts, provide opportunities for increased access to mental health care, but advocates must engage throughout the process to ensure consumers' needs are met. This article describes the advocacy experiences of the Mental Health Association of Maryland (MHAMD) and provides a historical perspective for current advocacy efforts. It discusses current health care reform initiatives in Maryland, similar to other states' efforts, and highlights critical issues of concern for advocates. Using examples from MHAMD's recent experience, 7 effective advocacy strategies are illustrated.*

At no time in our lives has consumer health care advocacy been more urgently needed, yet the general public remains remarkably disengaged in the generational shift that is now occurring in the structure of our health care system. This is not to say that consumer advocacy organizations have not played a central role in the legislative and regulatory arenas to protect the rights and interests of the general public. However, as reform plays out in states across the country, planning and implementation meetings are dominated by the businesses of health care rather than the end users of the system, despite the fact that the new architecture of the U.S. health system will impact the lives of each and every one of us, and our offspring, for generations to come.

In this article we explore the efforts of a mental health advocacy organization in one state to play a meaningful role in protecting the public interest, examining the key elements that have enabled consumer advocates to influence decision making. Exploring the issue of consumer involvement from the vantage point of mental health makes sense, as disability advocates have played a pivotal role for decades in impacting health and mental health policy. This is not surprising given the central role that these services play in the lives of individuals living with disabilities.

A brief overview of Maryland's rich history in mental health advocacy will be presented, as well as a snapshot of health care reform underway in the state, followed by a discussion of consumer advocacy efforts and their impact in influencing policy decisions.

## ADVOCACY LANDSCAPE

Maryland has a lengthy history of citizen mental health advocacy. The Mental Health Association of Maryland (MHAMD), one of the oldest mental health advocacy groups in the nation, was formed in 1915 and has long played a central role in coalition building to impact mental health policy.[1] Collaborative efforts began in the early 1980s with the founding of the Coalition for Citizens with Long-Term Mental Illnesses, which brought together MHAMD, the Maryland Association of Psychiatric Support Services (today the Community Behavioral Health Association of Maryland), National Alliance on Mental Illness (NAMI) Maryland and On Our Own of Maryland. These groups united to advance a unified policy agenda to improve access to quality mental health treatment.

Unity produced results, including passage of a Patient's Bill of Rights and successful budget initiatives to strengthen the community mental health system in the state. Moving into the 1990s, efforts expanded, as did the Coalition. One of the first state mental health parity bills in the nation was enacted in 1993, followed by a carve out in 1998 of mental health services from the state's 1115 Medicaid waiver. Both resulted from the efforts of a broad and growing coalition now known as the Maryland Behavioral Health Coalition, chaired by MHAMD. Member organizations included mental health consumers and family and advocacy groups, as well as mental health professional organizations, community mental health providers, and inpatient providers.

As successes occurred, so did sophistication of the network. Involvement in broader areas of policy resulted and offshoot networks developed. The Maryland Coalition on Mental Health and Aging formed in the late 1990s and the Mental Health and Criminal Justice Partnership first convened in 2005, both led by MHAMD and formed to focus attention on these discrete policy areas. During the same time period, child and adolescent issues received similar attention through formal and ad hoc coalition efforts. With a membership and volunteer base of consumers, family members, advocates, and providers, MHAMD has been uniquely positioned to broker consensus among the various mental health interests. Key to the collective success of these various networks has been a central and unwavering focus on the needs of individuals served by the public and private mental health systems.

## HEALTH REFORM IN MARYLAND

Maryland moved quickly after passage of the Patient Protection and Affordable Care Act (ACA) to become one of the landmark federal law's early adopters. A public process with broad opportunities for community participation has been a hallmark of Maryland's implementation effort. A 2010 Governor's Executive Order created a Health Care Reform Coordinating Council (HCRCC), which convened six subcommittees on various aspects of reform and issued recommendations in January 2011. Legislation to conform Maryland law to the ACA, establishment of the Governor's Office of Health Care Reform, and the Health Benefit Exchange Acts of 2011, 2012, and 2013 soon followed. In the 3 years since passage of the ACA, Maryland has formed many implementation committees to address issues such as health care delivery reform, exchange financing, outreach and education, essential health benefit selection, and health disparities.

The Health Benefit Exchange Act of 2011 established Maryland's Health Benefit Exchange and required various studies, resulting in the formation of advisory committees on plan management, continuity of care, the navigator program, exchange implementation, and financing and sustainability. Subsequently, the Health Benefit Exchange Act of 2012 established the Health Benefit Exchange Navigator Program, the mechanism to assist consumers with enrollment. Finally, in 2013 the Maryland Health Progress Act codified Medicaid expansion and provides continuity of care protections for individuals who transition between health insurance plans, including Medicaid.

## Behavioral Health Integration

In lock step with federal health care reform, states across the country are embarking on generational change in public mental health and substance use disorder service delivery, and Maryland is no exception. Efforts in our state seek to go beyond long planned for, yet scarcely implemented, efforts to integrate mental health and addiction treatment, through the inclusion of a central focus on somatic and behavioral health integration. Implementation is underway to merge two currently distinct state agencies for mental health and addiction treatment services, and regulations governing service providers in both disciplines will soon be conformed.

A broadly inclusive public process has occurred over the past two years to recommend a fiscal structure to integrate behavioral health and somatic services within the Medicaid program system. A recommendation resulting from this process was released in October 2012 and called for expansion of Maryland's mental health services carve-out to include substance use treatment services (currently delivered within a capitated Managed Care Organization [MCO] system). The Department of Health and Mental Hygiene approved this recommendation in April 2013 and launched an implementation phase with broad stakeholder involvement in June. An expansion of a request for proposals (RFP) to expand the role of the system's administrative services organization (ASO), addition of performance risk and shared savings within the ASO managed system, selection of outcome measures, and alignment of ASO and MCO obligations are the next steps in this process.

## Federal Parity Implementation

With all eyes focused on the passage of the ACA in 2010, implementation of the historic federal Mental Health Parity and Addiction Equity Act of 2008 began without much fanfare in 2010 once interim final regulations (IFR) were promulgated. It quickly became apparent that the IFR lacked clarity in some areas, making enforcement of the law difficult. Advocates worked tirelessly for the next 3 years impressing upon regulators the need for a timely release of final regulations with more specificity. In November 2013, 5 years since the passage of the historic law, final regulations that upheld and clarified the strong consumer protections in the IFR were promulgated. Attention now turns to enforcement of the law. In order to eradicate long-standing discriminatory practices that persist in the new insurance markets and ensure that the millions of newly insured will have access to the behavioral health care Congress intended, state insurance commissioners and federal enforcement agencies must take a proactive approach to enforcement.

## THE ROLE OF CONSUMER ADVOCATES

With the mind-numbing list of health reform committees and subcommittees underway over the past several years, one can imagine the near panic of mental health advocates in keeping up with this dizzying pace of activity to ensure that behavioral health concerns are not lost in the shuffle. Maryland is fortunate to have a strong citizen advocacy coalition focused on health care reform implementation, the Maryland Women's Coalition for Health Care Reform, which was formed in 2006. Alliance with this network of advocates proved essential to our success in advancing mutual goals. Seven principles, we call the seven Cs of effective advocacy, have guided our efforts and are summarized next.

## Content

For MHAMD, participating in various reform implementation committees and partnering with key allies were essential components of our successful effort. Being at the table from the start, becoming informed, and sharing useful information enabled us to be seen as an external stakeholder organization with something to offer. This was evidenced by the inclusion of MHAMD in the HCRCC's 2011 Health Care Reform Implementation Report, appointment to the HCRCC Communications and Outreach Committee, and the selection of MHAMD staff to serve on the Plan Management Advisory Committee, a post that enables us to directly impact the establishment of policies that will guide Maryland's Health Benefit Exchange.

Very few Behavioral Health Coalition members had time to devote to the plethora of health care reform implementation committees and meetings at the state level. We expanded the impact of our participation by keeping members informed and involved through meetings, e-mails, alerts, and blog posts. Drafting coalition letters on key issues of concern provided an easy way for mental health providers and advocates to make their voices heard.

The message regarding content is simple: Know your stuff. Be inquisitive and informed. Establish your credibility as a valued external partner by taking the time to gather and analyze data from a wide range of sources and bring useful knowledge to the table.

## Collaborate, Collaborate, Collaborate

Collaboration and coalition building have been, without question, the most important elements of our success in influencing health care reform implementation. Through the Behavioral Health Coalition, the Women's Coalition, and other networking forums, we have been able to expand our knowledge base and reach. Informal relationships across these groups have assisted all of us in covering meetings for each other, a small but critical building block that has enabled us to stay involved, share information, and coordinate strategy.

MHAMD was part of a diverse group of nontraditional allies in January 2012 when somatic health care advocates, consumer protection groups, health care providers, and insurance companies were able to put aside their differences and support the Maryland Health Benefit Exchange Act of 2012. Although not all stakeholders supported every tenet of the bill, all were able to support the larger intent, and no opposition to the bill was large enough to defeat it. Once the bill seemed destined for passage, the Behavioral Health Coalition partnered with somatic advocates to support specific amendments establishing important consumer protections, including mental health parity compliance language. This alliance ensured that behavioral health amendments were put forward as priorities from a broad stakeholder group, not just from behavioral health interests. Given the difficulty of gaining attention for behavioral health concerns in the massive reform effort underway, the importance of forging these relationships cannot be overstated.

The ACA requires that each state select essential health benefits that meet minimum federal standards, including compliance with the federal parity law. These essential benefits must be included in the qualified health plans that will be sold through health benefit exchanges, new insurance marketplaces to be established in each state where individuals and small businesses can secure affordable coverage. Led by the Maryland Women's Coalition, consumer advocates mounted a campaign for adoption of the State Employee Plan as Maryland's essential health benefit package, because it provides the most comprehensive array of basic coverage, including the most robust package of mental health and addiction treatment coverage among the possible offerings, but ultimately the Committee selected the largest small employer plan. Maryland's decision to select a small employer plan as the benchmark was a disappointment, but behavioral health and somatic advocates rallied in unison to reverse some effects of this course, ultimately securing substitution of the richer mental health and substance use disorder benefit in the federal Government Employees Health Association (GEHA) plan. Decision makers were swayed by the argument that bringing the non-parity-compliant small employer plan into compliance would be more difficult and costly than swapping for the parity-compliant plan in the initial phase. Building on our success in securing protections in the 2012 Exchange bill, relationships between somatic and behavioral health advocates further solidified.

Another challenge addressed through this growing collaboration was influencing Maryland Health Benefit Exchange plans to roll out Maryland's navigator program, which Congressional leaders wisely incorporated into the ACA to ensure that hard-to-reach populations would be made aware of new insurance opportunities available to them. Initially, siting this responsibility with insurance brokers or contracting this function out to a single vendor were proposed as implementation options. However, consumer advocates prevailed in securing a community-based approach that would better meet the public's needs, knowing that the very populations Congress sought to protect could best be served by local organizations already embedded in communities across the state. MHAMD joined with a growing network of coalition partners to support amendments to the 2012 Health Benefit Exchange bill to remove requirements that navigators be licensed insurance producers (brokers), while requiring a robust training standard for individual navigators that was appropriate to the task at hand.

As seasoned grassroots operators, we have been mindful of the importance of strength in numbers, and have worked continually to expand

Coalition participation. Expansion efforts have focused on both traditional and nontraditional partners. Testimony by the local chief of police or the CEO of a community hospital about unintended consequences of proposed mental health budget reductions can make even the most seasoned elected official take notice. Similarly, direct stories about real impact on individual constituents are critical. Through partnerships and joint projects with other organizations, including the Substance Abuse and Mental Health Services Administration (SAMHSA)-sponsored Health Care Reform Collaborative, we have built and leveraged relationships to bring these voices to the table.

These efforts played a central role in the final behavioral health integration recommendation endorsed by the state Health Department. A draft report was released by the state Health Department on behavioral health integration in September 2012. Although it contained many positive elements, mental health advocates had a few significant concerns. Through the Behavioral Health Coalition, we came together, identified key concerns, and sought broad community endorsement of a joint position statement, an effort that yielded 100 organizational signers. The next iteration of the report, released in October, reversed course and adopted the changes we had proposed. Although many factors could well have influenced this change, our ability to rally the troops at this critical moment would not have been possible without strong partnerships already in place.

The preceding examples reinforce the key elements of our collaborative strategies: networking far and wide, with traditional and nontraditional partners, and thinking strategically about who our allies are, including those who come to an issue from an entirely different vantage point. We strengthened our base by working in partnership to share the load, learned from the shared expertise around the table, and utilized a widened network of key contacts as our coalition grew. Rather than the outcome of the efforts of any one organization alone, our progress has truly been the result of the collective partnership of many organizations who share the common goal of improving health outcomes for the public.

## Clearly Define Goals

In the not-for-profit world, we are constantly bombarded with too much to do, too little time, too little staff, and too few resources. As mental health advocates have become more sophisticated, the range of issues within our purview has increased exponentially: child, adult and elderly concerns, criminal justice, education, housing, and the like compete for attention on our overloaded health policy plate. With this landscape in mind, it is essential to prioritize and stay focused on a limited agenda, on which sustained effort is most likely to yield progress that will positively impact core goals. As we plan strategically in our various coalitions, we routinely revisit and assess our priorities and progress, ensuring that we remain focused on the outcomes we are trying to achieve for the public.

## Communicate

A group of advocates comes together with a clearly defined goal. They seek to broaden their base of support. What is necessary to get there and what role does communication play?

First is the importance of message. No one wants to invest time without a clear sense of purpose and goals. But this alone is not enough. The ability to listen to partners and adapt in response to shared knowledge and concerns is paramount. As the Maryland Behavioral Health Coalition has grown and broadened its network, it has been critical to listen and learn from both traditional and nontraditional partners. Everyone's voice matters. Taking the time to seek input from a partner who comes to an issue from a completely different vantage point strengthens the group and its overall message. For years we have worked with substance use disorder treatment advocates on joint policy concerns with respect to care integration. This partnership has continued with the state's behavioral health integration effort. As differences emerged between mental health and substance use disorder treatment providers regarding the fiscal model for the system, our communication and collaboration skills were put to the test. Maintaining a focus on clinical issues, on which we do agree, has provided a path to continue in a collaborative spirit, despite differences regarding system structure.

Knowing that proper implementation of federal parity is essential to realizing equity in the treatment of behavioral health conditions, MHAMD endeavored to play a key role in ensuring the federal law's implementation. As one of the first states to enact mental health parity legislation in 1993, we were well aware of the pitfalls encountered by the public in seeking the coverage to which individuals were entitled. We decided the best route to assure federal parity was to implement a broadly focused communication campaign to educate consumers and providers about their new rights using traditional media, web, social marketing, and community outreach strategies. Additionally, knowing that the time commitment to move through the appeals process is a barrier for both consumers and providers, we decided to provide direct case assistance to individuals, in addition to a toolkit on how to file insurance complaints. These efforts have resulted in reimbursement for services that had been denied and changes to insurance plans that were not parity compliant. On a systems level, our experience through the Maryland Parity Project, funded by private foundations, has informed our efforts to impact health care reform discussions, and enabled us to provide real examples that influenced essential health benefit selection and implementation, qualified health plan certification and management, and continuity of care policies.

## Consensus

The Maryland Behavioral Health Coalition has always employed a consensus style in making decisions. Position statements are vetted through the group and modified in accord with our consumer-focused mission to build the broadest network of support possible. On the vast majority of issues, the network is in widespread agreement.

The scale of comprehensive system restructuring engenders anxiety and insular thinking in all of us. It is difficult to muster enthusiasm for a policy change that we know is best for the public, when its implementation could very well put the organization we run in the red, or worse, out of business. What is good for one segment of our advocacy network might be devastating for another branch. We have navigated these harsh realities through the use of a clearly defined decision-making process, one that is time consuming but well worth the extra effort. Major issues are discussed and debated at our regularly scheduled meetings. When Coalition members agree to adopt a joint position statement, the draft document goes out to the entire network for review and comment, often more than once. The final statement is sent to the entire network for signature. Only those groups who affirmatively choose to sign are listed, and we take the time to contact member organizations individually. This enables us to clearly understand the concerns of those who opt out. Because we do not send out position statements under a blanket letterhead and always include organizational names, our network is assured that we will not speak on their behalf without their explicit instruction.

## Consult and Compromise

Like building consensus, the process of compromise is not always quick or easy. Our position statement on behavioral health integration went through seven drafts before the final document was approved. Consulting, listening, and compromising over a period of months led to a product that was remarkably different from earlier drafts, but represented the broadest platform on which consensus could be built, with 63 organizations signing the final document. Subsequent communications with government leaders brought an ever-expanding network on board in support of our unified position, with 100 organizational cosigners ultimately secured.

Our Coalition has achieved notable success through a similarly collaborative demeanor and willingness to consult and compromise with government partners. We understand that change happens over time and recognize that in many instances incremental progress serves the public better than a hard-line combative stance that results in no movement at all. Through frequent formal and informal communication with government leaders, we strive to take the time to understand the broad political and budgetary realities within which they are working and recognize that our issues fit into a much broader framework of policy concerns that government officials are tasked with solving in economically trying times.

## Character

If there is one characteristic that we hope our work will be remembered by, it is integrity. We have always strived to be honest and fair in the conduct of business. A reputation builds over time and can easily be undone when inaccurate or false information is shared, partnerships are not respected, or relationships are undercut. Recently we were contacted by staff of the Maryland Health Benefit Exchange seeking to convene an ongoing group of mental health and substance use advocates to share our collective concerns. This suggests that we have evidenced understanding of the key issues, communicated well, shown strength in numbers, and presented ourselves as partners who deal honestly and are able to navigate to a consensus position. All of the qualities summarized in this article have played an important role in ensuring our effective participation as key stakeholders in a rapidly changing health care arena.

With a strong track record of involvement in reform, we will continue to navigate the waters ahead in dealing with upcoming issues such as strengthening provider network adequacy standards, assuring execution of continuity of care provisions for individuals moving between health plans, and implementation of parity and behavioral health integration.

## NOTE

1. To learn more about the Mental Health Association of Maryland and the Maryland Mental Health Coalition, visit www.mhamd.org.

# Behavioral Health Parity and the Affordable Care Act

### RICHARD G. FRANK

*Department of Health Care Policy, Harvard Medical School,*
*Boston, Massachusetts, USA*

### KIRSTEN BERONIO

*Office of Assistant Secretary for Planning & Evaluation, U.S. Department of Health and*
*Human Services, Washington, District of Columbia, USA*

### SHERRY A. GLIED

*Mailman School of Public Health, Columbia University, New York,*
*New York, USA*

*Prior to the passage of the Mental Health Parity and Addiction Equity Act (MHPAEA) and the Patient Protection and Affordable Care Act (ACA), about 49 million Americans were uninsured. Among those with employer-sponsored health insurance, 2% had coverage that entirely excluded mental health benefits and 7% had coverage that entirely excluded substance use treatment benefits. The rates of noncoverage for mental and substance use disorder care in the individual health insurance markets are considerably higher. Private health insurance generally limits the extent of these benefits. The combination of MHPEA and ACA extended overall health insurance coverage to more people and expanded the scope of coverage to include mental health and substance abuse benefits.*

On October 3, 2008, Congress enacted the Paul Wellstone and Pete Domenici Mental Health Parity and Addictions Equity Act (MHPAEA) (2008). MHPAEA extended the Mental Health Parity Act of 1996, which had prohibited the use of aggregate lifetime and annual dollar limits for mental health benefits in private insurance plans. Regulations implementing MHPAEA were published on February 2, 2010. A month later, the Patient Protection and Affordable Care Act (ACA) was enacted. In combination, these two laws serve to fundamentally alter the terms under which care for mental and substance use disorders are paid for in the United States. In this article, we describe how these two laws interact and affect insurance coverage for tens of millions of Americans.

In 2009, prior to the passage of MHPAEA and the Patient Protection and Affordable Care Act (2013) (known as the ACA) about 49 million Americans were uninsured (Garfield, Lave, & Donohue, 2010). Among those with employer-sponsored health insurance, 2% had coverage that entirely excluded mental health benefits and 7% had coverage that entirely excluded substance use treatment benefits. The rates of noncoverage for mental and substance use disorder care in the individual health insurance markets are considerably higher. Private health insurance that included mental health or substance use benefits generally limited the extent of these benefits. The combination of the MHPEA and the ACA extended overall health insurance coverage to more people, expanded the scope of coverage to include mental health and substance abuse benefits, and improved the coverage provided through those benefits (Bureau of Labor Statistics, 2012).

This article is organized into four sections. In the first section, we review the provisions of MHPAEA and explain how it affects coverage under large group insurance plans. We also discuss what the MHPAEA does not do and the segments of the insurance market that are not affected. The second section of the article explains the structure of coverage expansion provisions of the ACA. We focus first on private insurance coverage. This includes a review of the key elements of health insurance reform, including the individual mandate, the development of exchanges, the design of the essential health benefit (EHB), and the low-income subsidies that will enable people to afford coverage and care. This section also describes the expansion of coverage via Medicaid. In the third section of the article, we examine how the two laws interact and the quantitative impact of those interactions. The fourth and final section offers concluding observations.

## BACKGROUND ON THE MENTAL HEALTH PARITY AND ADDICTIONS EQUITY ACT

People with behavioral health problems (mental and substance use disorders) are disproportionately represented among the uninsured population (Substance Abuse and Mental Health Services Administration, 2010). Thus coverage expansion will potentially have an especially important impact on those with mental and substance use disorders. Prior to the implementation of MHPAEA in 2010, nearly two thirds of people with employer-sponsored coverage had special limits on inpatient behavioral health coverage and about three quarters faced limits on outpatient behavioral health coverage (Barry et al., 2003). About one quarter of those with employer-sponsored health insurance had coverage that required higher levels of cost sharing for behavioral health care. Thus prior to MHPAEA, the behavioral health coverage held by most privately insured Americans offered limited coverage of catastrophic expenses. The historical efficiency rationale for such limits involved concerns about excess costs or what is termed *moral hazard*. Yet in a world where private insurers and state Medicaid programs make extensive use of managed behavioral health care, there is abundant evidence showing that costs can be well controlled even alongside the types of coverage expansions spurred by parity for behavioral health care (Goldman, Frank, & Burnam, 2006).

## What Does Parity Require and What Does It Not Do?

The MHPAEA requires group insurers to ensure that the "financial requirements" and "treatment limitations" that are applicable to mental health and substance use benefits are no more restrictive than the predominant financial requirements and treatment limitations for medical and surgical benefits covered by the plan. The following simple summary highlights four key features of the MHPAEA.

1. The MHPAEA does not mandate coverage for mental and substance use disorder services. It only requires that financial requirements and treatment limitations are no more restrictive conditional on behavioral health services being covered.
2. The MHPAEA only addresses larger employer group insurance arrangements (those with 51 employees or more).
3. The MHPAEA regulates behavioral health insurance benefits by analogy. That is, the statute requires that coverage for behavioral health be judged against the standard of coverage for medical and surgical services.
4. It identifies a range of methods for rationing care that are used by health plans to limit use of services. These include copayments, coinsurance, and deductibles under the heading "financial requirements."

The law also refers to "limits on the frequency of treatment, number of visits, days of coverage or other similar limits on the scope or duration of treatment" in defining what must be no more restrictive (MHPAEA, 2008). This encompasses familiar benefit design parameters such as day and visit limits that have long been prevalent features of behavioral health coverage. It also pertains to management of behavioral health services that fall under "other similar limits on the scope and duration of treatment" (MHPAEA, 2008).

As noted, the statute explicitly recognizes that there are other ways to limit the "effective" level of coverage by using care management and other administrative mechanisms to ration care. Research has shown that care management can be applied to accomplish ends similar to results stemming from high copayments and strict treatment limits (Frank & McGuire, 2000). For this reason the MHPAEA regulations define what are termed *non-quantitative treatment limits* (NQTLs). NQTLs include medical management standards, prescription drug formulary structure, standards for including providers in a network, and methods for establishing fees, among other techniques. The regulations specify that a health plan may not impose an NQTL on mental health and substance use disorder services unless any processes, strategies, evidentiary standards, or other factors used to create the NQTL are comparable to and applied no more stringently for medical and surgical services. This means that the management of behavioral health care must be based on the same clinical and management processes used for management of medical and surgical care. This is complex to administer in practice, but it extended parity to all types of rationing mechanisms, which was clearly the intent of the statute.

At the time of this writing, final regulations have not been issued and thus there are some issues that were left unaddressed by the regulations issued in February 2010. Most significant were issues related to the scope of services. Key to setting out what is to be included in the scope of services is the way that certain analogous services are viewed. For example, in most medical and surgical coverage, so-called intermediate services are defined. They include postacute hospital care, postacute skilled nursing facility care, and home health care. In each case they are time limited (30–60 days). An important question for the final regulations is what the analogous services are in the behavioral health area. Some have proposed these to include partial hospital care, intensive outpatient care, and residential services.

## THE AFFORDABLE CARE ACT AND BEHAVIORAL HEALTH

The foundation of increased insurance coverage under the ACA is built on redesign and expansion of the small group and individual health insurance market and the expansion of Medicaid. The Congressional Budget Office (2013) estimates that the ACA will result in 37 million uninsured Americans gaining coverage. The ACA will expand coverage by providing subsidies for purchase of coverage in the nongroup market and expanded eligibility for Medicaid, and it will change the nature of coverage available in the nongroup and small-group markets.

### Private Insurance Expansion and Reform

The redesign of the small group and individual health insurance market consists of several key components. These include the individual mandate, low-income subsidies for premiums and cost sharing, the establishment of health insurance exchanges, and the definition of the EHBs.

*Private insurance subsidies* come in two forms, one for premiums and another for cost sharing. Individuals with incomes that are less than 400% of the federal poverty line (FPL) will be eligible for subsidies that defray premium costs and cost-sharing obligations. These subsidies are only available if the insurance is purchased through health insurance exchanges. The premium subsidy reduces premium costs through a tax credit. Subsidy levels are based on a sliding scale tied to income. The subsidy is also linked to a specific benefit design (the second lowest cost silver plan). Insurance sold through the exchanges also sets a cap on out-of-pocket costs for health care. This, too, varies with income level.

The *individual mandate* requires individuals to maintain "minimum essential coverage." Individuals who are permanent residents or citizens, have incomes that require filing a tax return ($9,350 for an individual and $18,700 for a family in 2010), and face out-of-pocket premium costs that amount to less than 8% of income must purchase health insurance or they can be assessed a tax penalty. The penalties are quite modest. In 2014, the penalty is $95 per adult and $47.50 per child or 1% of family income, whichever is greater. By 2016, they will be $695 per adult and $347.50 per child or 2.5% of family income, whichever is greater.

*Health insurance exchanges* reorganize the individual and small group health insurance market. Exchanges implement and enforce standards that certify health plans as "qualified" to sell health insurance through exchanges. To qualify for participation in the exchanges, health plans must meet EHB requirements and other marketing and quality requirements. For example, an exchange must ensure that a qualified health plan (QHP) offers a sufficient choice of providers. Issuers must be licensed and in good standing in each state in which coverage is offered. The term *good standing* means that the issuer has no outstanding sanctions imposed by a state's Department of Insurance.

Health plans must comply with quality improvement standards under the ACA. Plans can vary premiums for a QHP or multistate QHP by geographic rating area. Plans must charge the same premium rate for a plan, regardless of whether the plan is offered through the exchange, directly to a consumer, or through an agent. Health plans must cover all of the following groups using one or more combinations, including individuals, two-adult families, one-adult families with a child or children, and all other families.[1]

The EHB requirements govern the basic level of coverage. The ACA defines 10 components of coverage under the EHB that in effect define the mandated components of private insurance coverage. They include ambulatory services, emergency, hospitalization, maternity and newborn care, pediatric care, prescription drugs, preventive and wellness care, rehabilitative and habilitative and mental health and substance abuse care. The cost-sharing arrangements are set out in the statute under the bronze, silver, gold, and platinum options. The scope of services is defined by the typical private plan. Regulations have given states considerable discretion in choosing a benchmark for the EHB. The recent regulation governing the EHB allows states to choose among the following potential benchmark plans. They can select one of the three largest small group insurance plans in the state, the largest commercial health maintenance organization plan, one of the three largest health plans options for state employees, or one of the three largest plans that are part of the Federal Employees Health Benefit Program (see 45 CFR Parts 147, 155, and 156 [CMS-9980-P]. The rationale for this regulatory strategy is primarily twofold. First, because the coverage is aimed at individual and small group markets, using small group plans as a benchmark allows for a standard that is compatible with many small group plans. This is important because under the ACA, a state may require additional coverage beyond the EHB minimum for plans offered in the exchanges and in general, state laws governing small group and individual plans will apply to plans offered in the exchanges (as well as those offered outside the exchanges). However, states will have to cover the costs of any requirements beyond the EHB minimum. Second, health care varies dramatically across the country and some recognition of the heterogeneity of local conditions was seen as desirable. Several important implications stem from the reform of private health insurance markets.

One surprising finding is that only about 7% of the population under age 65 would be affected by the individual mandate provision in the ACA. This is a surprising finding given the rancor of the political debate around this provision of the law (Blumberg, Buettgens, & Feder, 2012). It is also important to recognize that the tax consequences of failing to adhere to the individual mandate are modest relative to the full cost of insurance. This means that the subsidies are likely to be the most important factor in affecting the level of program participation among people with incomes over 138% of the FPL (those above the Medicaid eligibility standard). Finally, the EHB provisions of the law mandate coverage of mental health and substance abuse services, which means that unlike MHPAEA, the ACA requires plans to cover care for mental and substance use disorders.

## Medicaid Expansion

The ACA creates a new mandatory eligibility group for Medicaid. It creates a simple income eligibility standard set at 133% of the FPL, with an additional 5% income allowance, effectively making the standard 138% of the FPL. This amounted to $15,415 and $26,344 for individuals and a family of three, respectively, in 2012. Meeting the income standard qualifies one for Medicaid regardless of other eligibility criteria for other categories; there is no asset test. The expansion is optional until 2014 and then is mandated. The

Supreme Court decision created a situation where there are no consequences of failing to implement the Medicaid expansion beyond foregoing federal subsidies for expansion. In effect, this makes expansion optional. The ACA creates enhanced federal funding for the Medicaid expansion. The federal government pays for 100% of the costs of the expansion in 2014 through 2016 and then phases down its participation to 90% by 2020.

The benefit design for those individuals newly covered under the Medicaid expansion will not necessarily be the states' existing Medicaid benefit structure. The statute outlines a number of benchmark plans that states may choose from in defining the coverage they will offer to the expansion group and the Center for Medicare and Medicaid Services (CMS) has clarified that states can use their Medicaid state plan as one option for defining the coverage they will provide. The CMS has adopted the term *alternative benefit plan* to refer to the coverage states could offer the expansion group. The ACA requires that the coverage states provide through these alternative benefit plans (ABPs) must comply with the EHB requirements and federal parity requirements to qualify for the enhanced match (see Proposed 42 CFR 440.315).

Following the admonitions in the ACA (Section 1937), the regulations allow states to design specialized benefit packages to address the special needs of target populations. Thus there may be different ABPs that apply to different population segments. The regulations also require that the full range of preventive services be included in the ABPs' coverage with no cost sharing. The regulations also allow for greater state flexibility in allowing cost sharing for services other than drugs, emergency room care, and preventive services. In the case of prescription drugs, greater flexibility is given to ABPs in creating tiered drug formularies.

The implications of the Medicaid expansion are several. A key result is that it is projected that roughly 65% of the newly covered people with mental and substance use disorders will be covered by the Medicaid expansion and Medicaid will become an even more significant source of coverage for people with mental health or substance use conditions (Donohue, Garfield, & Lave, 2010). A second implication is that because single childless adults will now be eligible for Medicaid, there will be many among the newly eligible with severe and persistent mental disorders who live in extreme poverty (less than 50% of the FPL), experience unstable housing, and have cooccurring substance use disorders. The flexibility provided to states under the ACA and through the regulations allows for the design of benefits that target the unique needs of people with significant impairments arising from serious and persistent mental illness.

## THE INTERACTION OF THE ACA AND MHPAEA

The ACA and MHPAEA interact in a number of very important ways that serve to greatly extend the reach of the MHPAEA legislation. In particular, the ACA legislation and the regulations that pertain to both the EHBs and ABPs require that benefit designs conform to the provisions of MHPAEA. The interaction between MHPAEA and the ACA operates through four channels. The inclusion of mental health and substance abuse services as one of the 10 required components of the EHB serves to mandate mental and substance use disorder coverage in both small group and individual private insurance (in and outside the exchanges) and in the Medicaid expansion coverage (all of which are subject to the EHB requirements under the ACA). The ACA also extended the MHPAEA requirements to qualified health plans, individual plans, and the coverage provided to the Medicaid expansion group. The regulations incorporated MHPAEA into the mental and substance use disorder components of the EHB. As a result, the requirement to cover mental and substance use disorder benefits in compliance with MHPAEA extends to small group and individual plans both inside and outside the exchanges. The rationale for this was to prevent the opportunity for less generous coverage outside the exchanges that would steer the better health care risks to plans outside the exchanges.

Together these features of the ACA and its implementation mean that MHPAEA protections are extended to small group and individual health insurance plans that were exempted from the MHPAEA provisions. Finally, the ACA and the proposed Medicaid expansion regulations state the MHPAEA provisions apply to the benefit designs of ABPs. Thus in combination, the four channels through which the ACA and MHPAEA interact mandate coverage at parity for all those gaining coverage through the exchanges and the Medicaid expansion, and extend parity requirements to existing plans in the small group and individual market.

## Estimated Impact

The quantitative implications of these interactions are profound, as summarized in Table 1. There are roughly 32 million people who currently do not have any insurance coverage for mental and substance use disorder care. Of that total, 5 million currently have health insurance coverage that does not cover mental and substance use disorder care. Those people benefit from the extension of MHPAEA to the individual and small group market. About 27 million people are currently uninsured and will gain coverage through either the exchanges or via the Medicaid expansion (as noted earlier, this is the lower end of the Congressional Budget Office impact estimate). That coverage will be at parity with medical and surgical coverage. In addition, another 30 million people who currently have private insurance coverage that includes mental and substance use disorder services through individual and small group plans will see their coverage for these services expanded. Thus a total of 62 million people will see a gain in coverage for mental and substance use disorder care as a result of the interaction of MHPAEA and the ACA.

**TABLE 1** Impact of Interactions of the Patient Protection and Affordable Care Act and Mental Health Parity and Addiction Equity Act

| | New coverage for mental and substance use disorder care | Expanded mental and substance use disorder care coverage | Total |
|---|---|---|---|
| Individuals currently holding individual coverage | 3.9 | 7.1 | 11 |
| Individuals currently with coverage under small group plans | 1.2 | 23.3 | 24.5 |
| Uninsured | 27 | — | 27 |
| Total | 32.1 | 30.4 | 62.5 |

*Note.* Data from Beronio, Po, Skopec, & Glied (2013).

In addition to offering individuals and households new financial protection against the financial consequences of needing mental and substance use disorder care, the ACA also offers important budgetary benefits to the states. As already noted, the federal government will pay for about 93% of the cost of the Medicaid expansion between 2014 and 2022 (Center on Budget and Priorities, 2012). Because states pay for public mental health systems that support people who are uninsured or underinsured for mental health care, the Medicaid expansion will offer states funds that would replace existing outlays from state general funds.

## Insurance and Financing Issues

MHPAEA regulates insurance and care management under health plans by analogy; that is, MHPAEA requires that the terms of coverage and care management for mental and substance use disorder care be no more restrictive than those for medical and surgical care. Thus the regulatory standards are based on a notion of comparability, and not on notions of clinical impact or financial risk protection that are typically at the heart of many benefit design considerations. This means that the binding constraints on mental and substance use disorder services include the scope of services for a medical and surgical benefit. For example, long-term care is typically not covered under private health insurance. Although many health plans cover postacute services like those in a skilled nursing facility or a rehabilitation hospital, these are typically of very limited time duration (e.g., 20–30 days). Thus, many treatments for severe mental and substance use disorders that require long-term services and supports (LTSS) that have been shown to be effective, like assertive community treatment, would not be required under MHPAEA.

The implication is that by setting a regulatory standard that depends on the structure of insurance for an analogous set of services, the coverage for mental and substance use disorders is only as comprehensive as the medical and surgical benefit. This fact is captured in Figure 1, which illustrates the

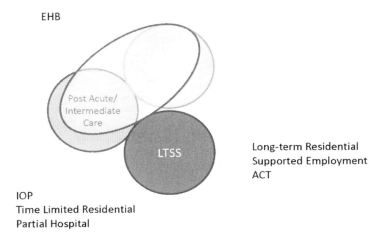

**FIGURE 1** What are the limits of coverage? EHB = essential health benefit; LTSS = long-term support services; ACT = assertive community treatment; IOP = intensive outpatient. (Color figure available online.)

potential gaps in coverage that might result from implementation of parity via the EHB and alternative health plan (AHP) coverage provisions in the ACA. Figure 1 highlights the fact that there will be a set of important services that are unlikely to be covered by many states' EHB and AHP benefit packages. So assertive community treatment, supported employment, supported housing, and long-term residential services are unlikely to be included in many state EHB and AHP designs.

The reality that there will be coverage gaps implies that paying for LTSS to meet the needs of low-income people with mental and substance user disorders will continue to make claims on state general funds and federal block grants. The recent recession has resulted in several years of declines in the budgets of state mental health programs. Many within and outside the federal government have begun to discuss the possibility of repurposing federal block grants used to pay for mental and substance use disorder services. Although it is clear that the coverage expansion of the ACA in the context of MHPAEA will direct new resources toward the care of people with mental and substance use disorders, it is equally clear that some important services for impaired low-income segments of the population will not be insured.

The confluence of the coverage expansion and the remnants of the budgetary impacts of the recession could have particular import for the supply of treatment for substance use disorders. The parity provisions in the ACA are especially significant for the coverage of care for substance use disorders (Buck, 2011). This is because people with these disorders are overrepresented among the uninsured, and coverage of substance use disorders in both Medicaid and private health insurance has been considerably more limited than even the mental health benefit. This means that one should expect significant increases in demand for substance use disorder treatment. However, because many of the services for this care have been financed by state grants and contracts, many of these providers have not had to meet the medical or administrative requirements for health care providers that bill private insurance and Medicaid. For this reason, there is a risk that at the very time that demand is expanding, the capacity to supply services will be less available. In fact it is estimated that close to 30% of substance use providers have never billed either Medicaid or private health insurance for services provided. The implication is that the combination of state cutbacks in support for substance use disorder care, coupled with the likelihood that a segment of existing providers will not qualify for reimbursement by public or private insurance, suggests potential shortages of providers for these services.

Finally, MHPAEA has been seen as a threat by segments of the managed behavioral health care (MBHC) industry. In fact several MBHC firms brought suit against the government when the MHPAEA regulations were issued. MHPAEA requires a close alignment of financial requirements, like deductibles, care management, and medical necessity criteria for mental and substance use disorder care and medical and surgical services. This is more difficult to accomplish under carve-out arrangements. The ACA, in addition to weaving MHPAEA into the fabric of health reform, also contains provisions with respect to delivery system reform that encourages integration of care for mental and substance use disorders with general medical care. Together these forces might force a shift in the carve-out model as it has evolved. Although the specialized expertise of the MBHC industry is clearly valued by purchasers, the need to better coordinate and integrate treatment for mental and substance use disorders and general medical care is seen as central to improving quality of care and making care more efficient. The carve-out model might further evolve to meet that need by adapting its care management systems to unify information and bolster communication between specialty mental and substance use disorder care and general medical care.


## CONCLUDING REMARKS

The enactment of Medicare and Medicaid served to fundamentally change the delivery of mental health care in the United States. It turned out to be far more powerful in driving mental health care changes than mental-health-specific policy efforts (Frank & Glied, 2006). The ACA drives new resources and financial protection toward mental and substance use disorder care. The intersection of the ACA and MHPAEA accomplish long-standing policy goals that date back to President John F. Kennedy. Like prior changes in payment and coverage, those brought about by the ACA will force important institutional change and will alter the roles of government agencies in overseeing the delivery of care. That is, mental and substance use disorder policy will become even more the purview of Medicaid and private insurance regulators than it is today. However, because coverage is necessarily incomplete, an important new policy challenge will be the continued financing of LTSS for people with mental and substance use disorder needs and the continued responsibility for true public health aspects like prevention and early intervention programs.

## FUNDING

The authors are grateful for the financial support of National Institute of Mental Health Grant R01 MH 094290.

## NOTE

1. Note that the ACA also prohibits preexisting condition exclusions for all Americans starting in 2014. It requires guaranteed issue and renewability in 2014. It decouples premiums from measures of health status in 2014. Lifetime caps on benefits were prohibited in September 2010 and annual limits are restricted and prohibited in 2014.

## REFERENCES

Barry, C. L., Gabel, J., Frank, R. G., Hawkins, S., Whitmore, H. H., & Pickreign, J. D. (2003). Design of mental health benefits: Still unequal after all these years. *Health Affairs, 22*(5), 127–137.

Beronio, K., Po, R., Skopec, L., & Glied, S. (2013). *Affordable Care Act expands mental health and substance use disorder benefits and federal parity protections for 62 million Americans* (ASPE Issue Brief). Washington, DC: U.S. Department of Health and Human Services.

Blumberg, L. J., Buettgens, M., & Feder, J. (2012). *The individual mandate in perspective.* Washington, DC: Urban Institute.

Buck, J. A. (2011). The looming expansion and transformation of public substance abuse treatment under the Affordable Care Act. *Health Affairs, 30*, 1402–1410.

Bureau of Labor Statistics. (2012). Unpublished tabulations from National Compensation Survey. Washington, DC: Department of Labor.

Center on Budget and Priorities. (2012). *How health reform's Medicaid expansion will impact state budgets.* Retrieved from http://www.cbpp.org/cms/index.cfm?fa=view&id=3801

Congressional Budget Office. (2013). *Effects of the Affordable Care Act on health insurance coverage.* Retrieved from http://www.cbo.gov/sites/default/files/cbofiles/attachments/03-13-Coverage%20Estimates.pdf

Donohue, J., Garfield, R., & Lave, J. (2010). *The impact of expanded health insurance coverage for individuals with mental illnesses and substance use disorders* (Report for the Assistant Secretary for Planning and Evaluation). Washington, DC: U.S. Department of Health and Human Services.

Frank, R. G., & Glied, S. A. (2006). *Better but not well: U.S. mental health policy since 1950*. Baltimore, MD: Johns Hopkins University Press.

Frank, R. G., & McGuire, T. G. (2000). Mental health. In A. Culyer & J. Newhouse (Eds.), *Handbook of health economics*, (pp. 893–954). Amsterdam, The Netherlands: North Holland.

Garfield, R. L., Lave, J. R., & Donohue, J. (2010). Health reform and scope of benefits for mental health and substance use disorder services. *Psychiatric Services, 61*, 1081–1086.

Goldman, H. H., Frank, R. G., & Burnam, M. A. (2006). Behavioral health parity for federal employees. *New England Journal of Medicine, 354*, 1378–1386.

Patient Protection and Affordable Care Act, HHS Notice of Benefit and Payment Parameters for 2012, 78 Fed. Reg. 1540 (March 11, 2013) (to be codified at 45 C.F.R. pts. 153, 155, 156, 157, & 158).

Mental Health Parity and Addictions Equity Act of 2008, Pub. L. No. 110–343 (2008).

Substance Abuse and Mental Health Services Administration. (2010). *National household survey on drug use and health*. Washington, DC: Author.

# The Affordable Care Act and Integrated Care

## FORD KURAMOTO

*Magna Systems, Inc., Los Angeles, California, USA*

*The Patient Protection and Affordable Care Act (ACA) of 2010 offers a comprehensive, integrated health insurance reform program for those who are eligible to enroll. A core feature of the ACA is the integration of primary health, behavioral health, and related services in a new national program for the first time. This article traces the history of past federal services integration efforts and identify varying approaches for implementing them to improve care, especially for underserved populations. The business case for integrated care, reducing escalating health care costs and overcoming barriers to implementation, is also discussed.*

Due to the passage of the Patient Protection and Affordable Care Act (ACA) in 2010 and its current process of implementation, many federal agencies, journalists, and experts have promulgated and published a great deal of information addressing the ACA. In some respects, the ACA culminates the evolution of federal health and human service coordination and integration efforts that began in the early 1930s. Consequently, addressing integrated care within the context of the ACA required the review of a substantial volume of print and electronic information, especially because the fields of primary health care, mental health, and substance use disorders each have their own specialized publications and literature. Identifying appropriate content for the discussion of integrated care from each of these three domains was a challenging task as some content issues were similar among the fields, but often the terms and concepts were slightly different. A major task involved collecting relevant information from many varied sources to define integrated care and discuss its importance to the ACA and its goals. To more clearly demonstrate differences and similarities, this report includes a significant number of tables and figures that contain pertinent information in a concise and detailed manner. These displays provide a wealth of useful concepts, examples, models, and reference material.

Much of this information and related literature focused on a primary health care perspective. However, for some time now, many in the field have endeavored to bring mental health and substance use disorder (SUD) services into closer working relationships with primary health services. Using a literature review of the history and current events on the integration of primary health, mental health, and SUD services pertinent to the ACA, this article addresses integrated care as a core feature of the ACA. The article discusses the definition of integrated behavioral health and primary health services, related organizational and service delivery issues, models and examples of integrated service programs, evidence of positive outcomes as a result of integrated services, barriers to implementation of integrated services, and the benefits of integrated services within the ACA.

The landmark ACA stands as perhaps the most important public health policy since the passage of the Medicare Act in 1965. The ACA will offer nearly 32 million uninsured Americans health insurance through the Medicaid expansion and other provisions. Historically, health care and behavioral health services were provided, often for the same patients, in separate service delivery systems without the needed integration. However, the ACA requires a set of comprehensive essential health benefits, establishes "health homes" wherein states can receive Medicaid support for providing integrated health services, provides for preventive services, encourages multidisciplinary teams, and addresses culturally competent services. The comprehensive provisions of the ACA explicitly create a national policy that integrates several aspects of health care, including a range of primary health care services from pediatrics to adult; outpatient and inpatient services; preventative, treatment, and rehabilitation services; mental health and SUD services; and behavioral health treatment. These comprehensive services are meant to be coordinated and integrated to foster quality care, for the best treatment outcomes as well as to reduce costs.

The following list includes a few examples of ways in which the provision of health and behavioral health services are related in terms of focusing on the patient's needs, although in separate service delivery systems:

- 10% to 20% of the general population will seek primary care services for a mental health problem (Van Egeren & Huber, n.d.).
- 66% of primary care patients with psychiatric diagnoses have significant physical illnesses.

- 50% to 66% of patients with psychiatric diagnoses go unrecognized by primary care providers.
- One study found that 60% of all medical visits were by "worried well" patients with no diagnosable disorder.
- Patients with mental health problems, compared to those without these issues, use twice the medical services.
- 33% to 50% of primary care patients refuse referrals to mental health professionals.
- Many patients prefer to receive mental health services within primary health care settings because they are not construed as "mental health care."
- 50% of all behavioral health disorders are treated in primary health care settings (Croghan & Brown, 2010).
- The annual medical expenses for chronic medical and behavioral health conditions combined cost 46% more than those with only a chronic medical condition.
- 70% of all primary health care visits have a psychosocial component (Bureau of Primary Health Care, n.d.).
- 90% of most common medical complaints have no organic basis.
- 48% of the appointments for all psychotropic drugs are with a nonpsychiatric primary care provider.
- 67% of psychoactive drugs are prescribed by primary care physicians.
- 80% of antidepressants are prescribed by primary care physicians.

These examples identify how primary health services interrelate with mental health and SUD services and affect clinical outcomes. Although these points do not directly address SUDs, they indicate that similar interrelatedness might apply to them, as well.


## HISTORICAL CONTEXT ON HUMAN SERVICES INTEGRATION

Major efforts to better organize government programs, and to reduce duplication, fragmentation, and costs began as early as 1932 with the Federal Committee on the Costs of Medical Care (Institute of Medicine [IOM] Board on Health Care Services, 1982). The committee found that fragmentation of care increased as specialization, increased number of federal grants, entitlements, and health programs became more complex. Adding to the complexity was the growth in different types of organizations and the size of government at the state and federal levels. Nearly 50 years after that 1932 study of medical care costs, the IOM studied the need for integrating health services and produced the report *Health Services Integration: Lessons for the 1980s*. This study investigated why some Americans did not always get the health care they needed or did not receive efficient or effective care.

The report concluded that the reasons were "fragmentation and gaps in the financing and provision of personal health services, especially for those with low incomes" (IOM Board on Health Care Services, 1982, p. 7) and the lack of integrated care. However, the political will to provide some form of comprehensive, integrated health care for all Americans did not come to fruition for nearly 80 years after the 1932 Federal Committee report and nearly 50 years after the development of Medicare until the passage of the ACA in 2010.

Note that the IOM study on health services integration discussed discrimination against ethnic minority populations. Although their case studies did not make an extensive effort to identify discrimination in the access and availability of services, they did find that few of the organizations studied had ethnic minority governing board members, even though their organizations served largely ethnic minority populations. This study did not place more emphasis on addressing racial discrimination, because the IOM Board of Health Care Services (1981) conducted another study at about the same time entitled *Health Care in a Context of Civil Rights*. Examples of how fragmentation and gaps in services occurred, especially for people with low incomes, include issues of eligibility for a variety of "categorical" services and trade-offs between costs and benefits (e.g., preventive services). The report found that services integration improved program efficiency and financial sustainability. The minimum integrated services recommended by this study included mental health care, preventive health services, and adequate nutrition for mothers and infants (IOM Board of Health Care Services, 1982).

Although progress toward the integration of mental health, SUDs, and primary health services slowly gained momentum, a few programs stand out as early leaders. One such program was the Eagleville Hospital, in Eagleville, PA. Started by the Jewish community as a tuberculosis sanitarium, the hospital has continuously operated for over 100 years to the present. In the 1960s, Eagleville Hospital started treating people with alcohol and other addictions and later developed one of the early cooccurring and integrated service programs about 1970 (Eagleville Hospital, n.d.). In 1966, the passage of the Comprehensive Health Planning and Public Health Services Act accelerated the movement toward health systems planning and integration.

By 1972, 56 states and territories established comprehensive health planning agencies and local jurisdictions established 158 area-wide agencies. These agencies improved the health of communities through health services planning and citizens' involvement. Residents of geographically defined communities (sometimes called *catchment areas*) were engaged in an open public process to improve the availability, accessibility, and quality of health care services as a means to improve the community's health status. Although these planning efforts emphasized consumer involvement as a core principle of the Federal Office of Economic Opportunity programs of the day, they included a focus on comprehensive and integrated services. For example, between 1996 and 2002, the W. K. Kellogg Foundation funded 41 local community partnerships in their Turning Point Program. This community engagement program defined public health concerns as having the following core functions:

- Community assets/mobilization;
- Health services for the underserved;
- Health services for the general population;
- Oral health;
- Behavioral health;
- Occupational health;
- Environmental health;
- Social determinants of health;
- Public safety;
- Economic development (Stern, 2008).

The federal government made grants available for comprehensive health planning at local and state levels. Many residents of the defined geographical communities and consumers of health services were engaged in this grassroots, community organizing process to improve health services. However, engaging consumers and giving them a voice in a well-intentioned health services planning process had its difficulties, in terms of improving the health status of a community. This was particularly true because the input of all of the stakeholders in a specified community focused only on health services planning and not on the operations of the service infrastructure. The health care providers, including solo practice physicians, health maintenance organizations (HMOs), nonprofit hospitals, and clinics, and health insurance carriers as part of the health care service delivery system were not the direct focus of comprehensive health planning (O'Connor, 1974). Finally, with the enactment of the ACA in 2010 the nation's public health policy engaged both consumers and providers in an integrated, comprehensive planning and implementation process to improve the health status of Americans at the local, state, and national levels.

## DEFINING INTEGRATED CARE AND IDENTIFYING VARIOUS FORMS OF INTEGRATION

Many different terms regarding various levels or types of services integration have emerged over the years. As previously discussed, as early as 1932, a federal committee noted that some form of integration was needed to reduce fragmentation and duplication of government health and human service programs. For example, one familiar form of collaboration between mental health and SUD services is for treating cooccurring disorders. They require treatment protocols involving both mental health and SUD services in a coordinated, collaborative manner. Other forms of integration include medical-provided behavioral health care, co-location, reverse co-location, and disease management (Collins, Levis Hewson, Munger, & Wadem, 2010). However, the most relevant forms of integration for this discussion involve the following:

- *Horizontal integration.* This is unified or coordinated delivery of the full range of health care services appropriate for a particular patient, usually involving the coordinated delivery of on-site services, although it might involve other organizations or providers (IOM Board on Health Care Services, 1982).
- *Vertical integration.* Vertical linkages are made between the primary care site and secondary, tertiary, and long-term care (IOM Board on Health Care Services, 1982).
- *Collaboration and the collaborative care model.* Collaboration is a model of professions working closely together in the delivery of care, but not subsumed into a single organizational framework. Collaboration is a pre-condition to integration (Boon, Mior, Barnsley, Ashbury, & Haig, 2009). The collaborative care model is an evidence-based approach to treating depression and chronic physical disease in a primary care setting. This model involves an on-site care manager and mental health consultants who are members of a primary care team (Unutzer, Harbin, Schoenbeum, & Druss, 2013).
- *Bidirectional integration.* This is integration of behavioral health and primary care services (SAMHSA–HRSA Center for Integrated Health Solutions, n.d.-a).

The Substance Abuse and Mental Health Services Administration (SAMHSA) defines the integration of health and behavioral health services as "the systematic coordination of general and behavioral healthcare. Integrating mental health, substance abuse and primary care services produces the best outcomes and proves the most effective approach to caring for people with multiple health care needs" (SAMHSA–HRSA Center for Integrated Health Solutions, n.d.-c).

The ACA legislation incorporates provisions from the Mental Health Parity and Addiction Equity Act of 2008 (MHPAEA), proposed by the late Senator Paul Wellstone (D-MN) and former Senator Pete Domenici (R-NM). With the inclusion of the MHPAEA, the 2010 ACA legislation made the integration of health and behavioral health services federal public health policy for the first time in U.S. history. The MPHAEA requires the coverage of mental health and SUD services at parity with primary health coverage. It specifically prohibits group health plans imposing more stringent treatment limitations and financial requirements for mental health and SUD services than for medical and surgical benefits.

Based on studies in the literature, Table 1 provides a series of definitions of integration as well as collaborative care. Note that the studies listed in Table 1 mention mental health issues, but do not specifically include SUDs.

As previously discussed, existing literature regarding the integration of health and behavioral health services includes varying points of view regarding what integration means and how to plan and implement effective programs. Consequently, integration to maximize treatment outcomes and provide sustainable, financially viable services among diverse service providers could take differing forms among the states. Various models of health and behavioral health services collaboration help clarify these approaches.

Van Egeren and Huber (n.d.) developed a three-level model of collaboration among primary health care and behavioral health services shown here to help clarify the characteristics of each:

Level 1: Minimal collaboration—Providers in separate locations
- Separate systems.
- Rarely communicate about patients.
- Most private practices and agencies.
- Handles adequately problems with little biopsychosocial interplay and few management difficulties.
- Handles inadequately problems that are refractory to treatment or have significant biopsychosocial interplay.

Level 2: Basic collaboration on site
- Separate systems but share same facility.
- No systematic approach to collaboration—do not share common language or in-depth understanding of each other's worlds—misunderstandings are common.
- Common in HMO settings.
- Handles adequately problems with moderate biopsychosocial interplay requiring occasional communication about shared patients.
- Handles inadequately patients with ongoing and challenging management problems.

Level 3: Close collaboration in fully integrated system
- Same site, same vision, and same system in a seamless web of biopsychosocial services.
    1. Staff committed to biopsychosocial systems paradigm.
    2. In-depth understanding of each other's roles and cultures.
    3. Operates as a team—regular collaboration.
- Fairly rare. Occurs in some hospice centers and special training and clinical settings.
- Handles adequately most difficult and complex biopsychosocial problems with challenging management problems.
- Handles inadequately problems when resources of health care team are insufficient or when there is breakdown with larger service system.

THE AFFORDABLE CARE ACT AND INTEGRATED BEHAVIORAL HEALTH CARE

**TABLE 1** Definitions of Clinically Integrated Health Care

| Source | Definition of integration |
| --- | --- |
| Institute of Medicine (2006) | Integrated treatment: "refers to interactions between clinicians to address the individual needs of the client/patient" and consists of "any mechanism by which treatment interventions for co-occurring disorders are combined within the context of a primary treatment relationship or service setting" (see p. 213). |
| Shortell (2000) | Clinical integration: "extent to which patient care services are coordinated across people, functions, activities, and sites over time so as to maximize the value of the services delivered to the patient." |
| Strosahl (1998, as reported in Robinson & Reiter, 2007) | Integration: "integration occurs when the mental health provider is considered a regular part of the health care team." |
| Blount (2003, pp. 122, 124) | Integrated services "have medical and behavioral health components within one treatment plan for a specific patient or population of patients." Integrated care "describes care in which there is one treatment plan with behavioral and medical elements rather than two treatment plans. The treatment plan is delivered by a team that works together very closely or by pre-arranged protocol." |
| Byrd et al. (2005, p. 2) | Integrated care: "the process and product of medical and mental health professionals working collaboratively and coherently toward optimizing patient health through biopsychosocial modes of prevention and intervention." |
| Veterans Administration (2005) | Integrated behavioral model "is to support the primary care provider in identifying and treating patients with mental health diagnoses and/or need for behavioral interventions." |
| Smith (2007) | Integrated care: "recognized by the acceptance of one individual clinician of responsibility for assessment, planning, linking, monitoring, advocacy, and outreach with respect to all factors that are pertinent to meeting an individual's health care needs and achieving cost-effectiveness outcomes." |
| Hogg Foundation (2008) | Integrated health care approach: "primary care and mental health providers partner to manage the treatment of mental health problems in the primary care or pediatric setting and to address barriers to implementation that they encounter." |
| American Psychological Association, Presidential Task Force on Integrated Health Care for an Aging Population (2008, p. 21) | Integrated health care: "characterized by a high degree of collaboration among the various health professionals servicing patients in terms of assessment, treatment planning, treatment implementation, and outcome evaluation." |

| Source | Definition of collaborative care |
| --- | --- |
| Bower (2006) | Collaborative care: a multifaceted organizational intervention, which could include a number of components: (a) the introduction of a new role (case manager) into primary care, to assist in the management of patients with depression through structured and systematic delivery of interventions; (b) the introduction of mechanisms to foster closer liaison |

*(Continued)*

**TABLE 1** Continued

| Source | Definition of collaborative care |
|---|---|
|  | between primary care clinicians and mental health specialists (including case managers) around individual patient care; (c) the introduction of mechanisms to collect and share information on the progress of individual patients. |
| Katon (2003) | Collaborative care is a multimodal intervention that includes integration of a care manager into primary care who works with both patient and PCP and helps with developing a shared definition of the problem, providing patient education and support, developing a shared focus on specific problems, targeting goals and a specific action plan, offering support and problem solving to optimize self-management, achieving closer monitoring of adherence and outcomes, and facilitating appointments to the PCP or specialist for patients with adverse outcomes or side effects. |
| Gagne (2005), Canadian Collaborative Mental Health Initiative | Collaborative care is not a fixed model or specific approach; rather, it is a concept that emphasizes the opportunities to strengthen the accessibility and delivery of mental health services through primary health care settings through interdisciplinary collaboration. |

*Note.* PCP = primary care provider. *Source*: Butler et al. (2008).

Figure 1 illustrates the relationships among the service activities and entities including integrated service providers and patients in a fairly complete integrated care system.

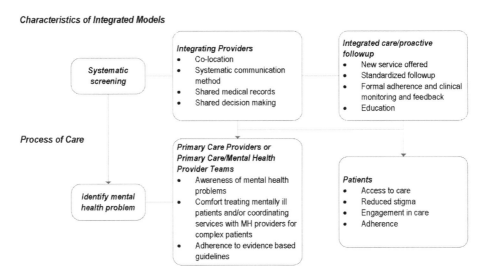

**FIGURE 1** Characteristics of integration linked to process of care. MH = mental health. *Source*: Butler et al. (2008).

## THE ACA ESSENTIAL HEALTH BENEFITS AND INTEGRATED CARE MODELS

This section focuses on the ACA and its integration of health care, mental health, and SUD services. The ACA essential health benefits created a holistic approach to the health care needs of an individual's mind and body that, for the first time, advances public health policy through the integration of primary health care and behavioral health services. The ACA lists 10 categories of essential health benefits required to offer high-quality, affordable health insurance to all enrollees. The ACA requires that at a minimum, states offer the following comprehensive services:

1. Ambulatory patient services;
2. Emergency services;
3. Hospitalization;
4. Maternity and newborn care;
5. Mental health and SUD services, including behavioral health treatment;
6. Prescription drugs;
7. Rehabilitative and habilitative services and devices;
8. Laboratory services;
9. Preventive and wellness services and chronic disease management;
10. Pediatric services, including oral and vision care.

Organizational cultures vary widely in their implementation of clinical practice and service programs. To integrate the behavioral health parity provisions into programs, organizations must address these variances. The Center for Integrated Health Solutions (CIHS), supported by SAMHSA and Health Resources and Services Administration (HRSA), identified five basic models of integration or ways to conceptualize integration:

- *Behavioral health homes.* A behavioral health home agency serves as a health home for people with mental health and SUD service needs. The model proposes a set of core clinical features of a behavioral health home.
- *The Primary and Behavioral Health Care Integration (PBHCI) Program.* Developed by SAMHSA, this program supports the expansion of integrated primary care services into publicly funded, community-based behavioral health settings. Since 2006, SAMHSA has awarded PBHCI grants to 94 organizations.
- *The four-quadrant model.* This model illustrates the relationships between the primary care and mental health and SUD complexities and risk factors (see Figure 2).
- *The mental health/primary care integration model.* This model illustrated in Table 2 includes comments regarding the relationships between it and the four-quadrant model.

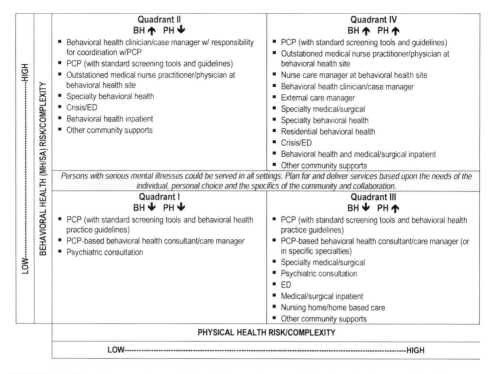

**FIGURE 2** The four-quadrant clinical integration model. BH = behavioral health; PH = physical health; PCP = primary care provider; ED = emergency department; MH/SA = mental mental health/substance abuse. *Source*: SAMHSA–HRSA Center for Integrated Health Solutions (n.d.-b).

- *The standard framework for levels of integrated health care.* CIHS produced this model to help organizations self-assess their progress on the continuum of integration (see Table 3 for the CIHS chart of the six levels of collaboration/integration core descriptions).

This CIHS list of examples includes the well-known four-quadrant clinical integration model (SAMHSA–HRSA Center for Integrated Health Solutions, n.d.-b). Figure 2 helps conceptualize how integration might be bidirectional in the quadrants that indicate differing levels of integration.

The four-quadrant model divides the general treatment population into four groups based on their behavioral and physical health risk and status. The model then suggests service elements to address the needs of each particular subpopulation. The quadrants in the four-quadrant model are characterized as follows.

- Quadrant I: Low behavioral and physical complexity or risk. Clients served in primary care with behavioral health staff on site.

**TABLE 2** Mental Health and Primary Care Levels of Integration Options

| Function | Minimal collaboration | Basic collaboration from a distance | Basic collaboration on-site | Close collaboration/ partly integrated | Fully integrated/ merged |
|---|---|---|---|---|---|
| The consumer and staff perspective/experience | | | | | |
| Access | Two front doors; consumers go to separate sites and organizations for services | Two front doors; cross-system conversations on individual cases with signed releases of information | Separate reception, but accessible at same site; easier collaboration at time of service | Same reception; some joint service provided with two providers with some overlap | One reception area where appointments are scheduled; usually one health record, one visit to address all needs; integrated provider model |
| Services | Separate and distinct services and treatment plans; two physicians prescribing | Separate and distinct services with occasional sharing of treatment plans for Q4 consumers | Two physicians prescribing with consultation; two treatment plans but routine sharing on individual plans, probably in all quadrants | Q1 and Q3 one physician prescribing, with consultation; Q2 and Q4 two physicians prescribing some treatment plan integration, but not consistently with all consumers | One treatment plan with all consumers, one site for all services; ongoing consultation and involvement in services; one physician prescribing for Q1, Q2, Q3, and some Q4; two physicians for some Q4: one set of lab work |
| Funding | Separate systems and funding sources, no sharing of resources | Separate funding systems; both may contribute to one project | Separate funding, but sharing of some on-site expenses | Separate funding with shared on-site expenses, shared staffing costs, and infrastructure | Integrated funding, with resources shared across needs; maximization of billing and support staff; potential new flexibility |

*(Continued)*

**TABLE 2** *Continued*

| Function | Minimal collaboration | Basic collaboration from a distance | Basic collaboration on-site | Close collaboration/ partly integrated | Fully integrated/ merged |
|---|---|---|---|---|---|
| Governance | Separate systems with little or no collaboration; consumer is left to navigate the chasm | Two governing boards; line staff work together on individual cases | Two governing boards with executive director collaboration on services for groups of consumers, probably Q4 | Two governing boards that meet together periodically to discuss mutual issues | One board with equal representation from each partner |
| EBP | Individual EBPs implemented in each system | Two providers, some sharing of information but responsibility for care cited in one clinic or the other | Some sharing of EBPs around high utilizers (Q4); some sharing of knowledge across disciplines | Sharing of EBPs across systems; joint monitoring of health conditions for more quadrants | EBPs like PHQ-9; IDDT, diabetes management; cardiac care provider across populations in all quadrants |
| Data | Separate systems, often paper based, little if any sharing of data | Separate data sets, some discussion with each other of what data shares | Separate data sets; some collaboration on individual cases | Separate data sets, some collaboration around some individual cases; maybe some aggregate data sharing on population groups | Fully integrated, (electronic) health record with information available to all practitioners on need to know basis; data collection from one source |

*Note.* EBP = evidence-based practice; PHQ-9 = Patient Health Questionnaire-9; IDDT = Integrated Dual Disorder Treatment. *Source*: SAMHSA-HRSA Center for Integrated Health Solutions (2006).

**TABLE 3** Six Levels of Collaboration/Integration

| Level 1: Minimal collaboration | Level 2: Basic collaboration at a distance | Level 3: Basic collaboration online | Level 4: Close collaboration onsite with some systems integration | Level 5: Close collaboration approaching an integrated practice | Level 6: Full collaboration in a transformed/ merged integrated practice |
|---|---|---|---|---|---|
| Core descriptions | | | | | |
| Coordinated key element: Communication | | Colocated key element: Physical proximity | | Integrated key element: Practice change | |
| Behavioral health, primary care, and other health care providers at work | | | | | |
| In separate facilities, where they:<br>• Have separate systems<br>• Communicate about cases only rarely and under compelling circumstances<br>• Communicate, driven by provider need<br>• Might never meet in person<br>• Have limited understanding of each other's roles | In separate facilities, where they:<br>• Have separate systems<br>• Communicate periodically about shared patients<br>• Communicate, driven by specific patient issues<br>• Might meet as part of larger community<br>• Appreciate each other's roles as resources | In same facility, not necessarily same offices, where they:<br>• Have separate systems<br>• Communicate regularly about shared patients, by phone or e-mail<br>• Collaborate, driven by need for each other's services and one reliable referral<br>• Meet occasionally to discuss cases due to close proximity<br>• Feel part of a larger yet ill-defined team | In same space within the same facility, where they:<br>• Share some systems, like scheduling or medical records<br>• Communicate in person as needed<br>• Collaborate, driven by need for consultation and coordinated plans for difficult patients<br>• Have regular face-to-face interactions about some patients<br>• Have a basic understanding of roles and culture | In same space within the same facility (some shared space), where they:<br>• Actively seek system solutions together or develop work-arounds<br>• Communicate frequently in person<br>• Collaborate, driven by desire to be a member of the care team<br>• Have regular team meetings to discuss overall patient care and specific patient issues<br>• Have an in-depth understanding of roles and culture | In same space within the same facility, sharing all practice space, where they:<br>• Have resolved most or all system issues, functioning as one integrated system<br>• Communicate consistently at the system, team, and individual levels<br>• Collaborate, driven by shared concept of team care<br>• Have formal and informal meetings to support integrated model of care<br>• Have roles and cultures that blur or blend |

(*Continued*)

**TABLE 3** Continued

| Key differentiators | | | | | |
|---|---|---|---|---|---|

**Clinical delivery**

- Screening and assessment done according to separate practice models
- Separate treatment plans
- Evidenced-based practices (EBPs) implemented separately

- Screening based on separate practices; information may be shared through formal requests or health information exchanges
- Separate treatment plans shared based on established relationships between specific providers
- Separate responsibility for care/EBPs

- May agree on a specific screening or other criteria for more effective in-house referral
- Separate service plans with some shared information that informs them
- Some shared knowledge of each other's EBPs, especially for high utilizers

- Agree on specific screening, based on ability to respond to results
- Collaborative treatment planning for specific patients
- Some EBPs and some training shared, focused on interest or specific population needs

- Consistent set of agreed on screenings across disciplines, which guide treatment interventions
- Collaborative treatment planning for all shared patients
- EBPs shared across system with some joint monitoring of health conditions for some patients

- Population-based medical and behavioral health screening is standard practice with results available to all and response protocols in place
- One treatment plan for all patients
- EBPs are team selected, trained, and implemented across disciplines as standard practice

**Patient experience**

- Patient physical and behavioral health needs are treated as separate issues
- Patients must negotiate separate practices and sites on their own with varying degrees of success

- Patient health needs are treated separately, but records are shared, promoting better provider knowledge
- Patients may be referred, but a variety of barriers prevent many patients from accessing care

- Patient health needs are treated separately at the same location
- Close proximity allows referrals to be more successful and easier for patients, although who gets referred might vary by provider

- Patient needs are treated separately at the same site, collaboration might include warm hand-offs to other treatment providers
- Patients are internally referred with better follow up, but collaboration might still be experienced as separate services

- Patient needs are treated as a team for shared patients (for those who screen positive on screening measures) and separately for others
- Care is responsive to identified patient needs by a team of providers as needed, which feels like a one-stop shop

- All patient health needs are treated for all patients by a team, who function effectively together
- Patients experience a seamless response to all health care needs as they present, in a unified practice

**Practice/organization**

| | | | | | |
|---|---|---|---|---|---|
| • No coordination or management of collaborative efforts<br>• Little provider buy-in to integration or even collaboration, up to individual providers to initiate as time and practice limits allow | • Some practice leadership in more systematic information sharing<br>• Some provider buy-in to collaboration and value placed on having needed information | • Organization leaders supportive but often colocation is viewed as a project or program<br>• Provider buy-in to making referrals work and appreciation of on-site availability | • Organization leaders support integration through mutual problem solving of some system barriers<br>• More buy-in to concept of integration but not consistent across providers, not all providers using opportunities for integration or components | • Organization leaders support integration, if funding allows and efforts placed in solving as many system issues as possible, without changing fundamentally how disciplines are practiced<br>• Nearly all providers engaged in integrated model. Buy-in might not include change in practice strategy for individual providers | • Organization leaders strongly support integration as practice model with expected change in service delivery, and resources provided for development<br>• Integrated care and all components embraced by all providers and active involvement in practice change |

**Business model**

| | | | | | |
|---|---|---|---|---|---|
| • Separate funding<br>• No sharing of resources<br>• Separate billing practices | • Separate funding<br>• Might share resources for single projects<br>• Separate billing practices | • Separate funding<br>• Might share facility expenses<br>• Separate billing practices | • Separate funding, but might share grants<br>• Might share office expenses, staffing costs, or infrastructure<br>• Separate billing due to system barriers | • Blended funding based on contracts, grants, or agreements<br>• Variety of ways to structure the sharing of all expenses<br>• Billing function combined or agreed on process | • Integrated funding, based on multiple sources of revenue<br>• Resources shared and allocated across whole practice<br>• Billing maximized for integrated model and single billing structure |

---

Advantages and weaknesses at each level of collaboration/integration

---

**Advantages**

| | | | | | |
|---|---|---|---|---|---|
| • Each practice can make timely and autonomous decisions about care | • Maintains each practice's basic operating structure, so change is not a | • Colocation allows for more direct interaction and communication among | • Removal of some system barriers, like separate records, allows closer collaboration to occur | • High level of collaboration leads to more responsive patient care, increasing | • Opportunity to truly treat whole person<br>• All or almost all system barriers resolved, allowing providers to |

---

(Continued)

**TABLE 3** Continued

Advantages and weaknesses at each level of collaboration/integration

| | | | | |
|---|---|---|---|---|
| • Readily understood as a practice model by patients and providers | …disruptive factor<br>• Provides some coordination and information-sharing that is helpful to both patients and providers | …professionals to impact patient care<br>• Referrals more successful due to proximity<br>• Opportunity to develop closer professional relationships | …engagement, and adherence to treatment plans<br>• Provider flexibility increases as system issues and barriers are resolved<br>• Both provider and patient satisfaction might increase | …practice as high-functioning team<br>• All patient needs addressed as they occur<br>• Shared knowledge base of providers increases and allows each professional to respond more broadly and adequately to any issue |
| **Weaknesses**<br>• Services might overlap, be duplicated, or even work against each other<br>• Important aspects of care might not be addressed or take a long time to be diagnosed | • Sharing of information might not be systematic enough to affect overall patient care<br>• No guarantee that information will change plan or strategy of each provider<br>• Referrals might fail due to barriers, leading to patient and provider frustration | • Proximity might not lead to greater collaboration, limiting value<br>• Effort is required to develop relationships<br>• Limited flexibility, if traditional roles are maintained | • System issues might limit collaboration<br>• Potential for tension and conflicting agendas among providers as practice boundaries loosen | • Practice changes might create lack of fit for some established providers<br>• Time is needed to collaborate at this high level and might affect practice productivity or cadence of care<br><br>• Sustainability issues might stress the practice<br>• Few models at this level with enough experience to support value<br>• Outcome expectations not yet established |

*Note. Source:* Heath, Wise Romero, and Reynolds (2013).

THE AFFORDABLE CARE ACT AND INTEGRATED BEHAVIORAL HEALTH CARE

- Quadrant II: High behavioral health, low physical health complexity or risk. Clients served in a specialty behavioral health system that coordinates with the primary care provider, or in more advanced integrated systems, that provides primary care services within the behavioral health setting.
- Quadrant III: Low behavioral, high physical health complexity or risk. Clients served in the primary care or medical specialty system with behavioral staff on site in primary or medical specialty care, coordinating with all medical care providers including disease care managers.
- Quadrant IV: High behavioral, high physical health complexity or risk. Clients served in both the specialty behavioral health and primary care or medical specialty systems (Mauer, 2006). (See the National Association of State Mental Health Program Directors, 2005, for a more detailed discussion of the four-quadrant model).

Further approaches to integration can also be viewed from the perspective of how behavioral staff is utilized, the identified target population to be served, and the levels and types of collaboration involved. Table 2 provides five levels of integration across six functions from the perspectives of both consumers and staff. Note that Table 2 also includes a discussion of the relationships among Figure 2, the four-quadrant model, and Table 2 levels of integration options.

Table 3, the six levels of collaboration/integration, by Heath, Wise Romero, and Reynolds (2013), provides an even more detailed analysis of six levels of collaboration and integration across five dimensions and "key differentiators." The five dimensions are behavioral health, primary care and other health care providers, clinical delivery, atient experience, practice organization, and business model. Table 3 concludes with a section on advantages and weaknesses at each level of collaboration or integration.

## SAMHSA Integration Programs

SAMHSA has placed a priority on efforts to transform health care in the United States. To accomplish this, SAMHSA has identified Strategic Initiative #5 as health reform and Goal 5.5 is to "Foster the integration of primary and behavioral healthcare." They clearly demonstrate SAMHSA's commitment to ACA and integrated services (SAMHSA, 2011). Additionally, SAMHSA provides technical assistance and training to promote the integration of primary and behavioral health care. SAMHSA collaborated with the HRSA to create the SAMHSA–HRSA CIHS for information and resources on the "bidirectional integration of behavioral health and primary care" (SAMHSA–HRSA Center for Integrated Health Solutions, n.d.-a). As previously mentioned, SAMHSA has also funded 94 PBHCI grants to community-based behavioral health organizations since 2006 to expand the number of local programs making the transition to fully integrated care that will be eligible for Medicaid and other reimbursements.

In 2003, SAMHSA initiated the Screening, Brief Intervention, and Referral to Treatment (SBIRT) program to promote services integration. Since 2003, SAMHSA has made grants to 15 single state agencies, 17 colleges and universities, medical residency programs, and 12 targeted capacity expansion campus screening and brief intervention grants (Office of National Drug Control Policy, 2012). The use of the SBIRT approach was expanded to primary health care settings when the Centers for Medicare and Medicaid Services made it possible for federally qualified health centers to receive reimbursements for SBIRT services beginning in 2005 (SAMHSA, 2012).

## Agency for Healthcare Research and Quality on Integration and Outcome Measures

The Agency for Healthcare Research and Quality (AHRQ) conducted research on the integration of primary and behavioral health care on patient outcomes and found that integration improved patient outcomes. For example, AHRQ reported on an extensive analysis of studies in the literature regarding various forms of integrated primary and behavioral health care services (Butler et al., 2008). This article identified the different types of integrated service delivery systems in the literature, which is a complicated task. Trying to measure the improvement in client outcomes, based on the specific type of integrated service system used, makes the task even more complicated. Nevertheless, this article concluded that in general, the integration of mental health, substance abuse, and primary care has a positive effect on client outcomes.

The article also raised several important issues that affect the potential success of integration, such as determining the "business case" for financing integration. It raised questions regarding how health plans and physician group practices will decide to handle the fiscal complexities of integrated care services financed by a new fee-for-service payment system. However, recent developments in financing through the ACA might offer new opportunities to address these issues, such as the Medicaid health home. Further, Unutzer and colleagues (2013) suggested that mental health specialists see only 20% of adult patients with mental health disorders. Many patients, whether they need to be seen by mental health specialists or not, generally prefer to be seen in primary care settings, where they feel less stigma. Primary-care-based Medicaid health homes, using the evidence-based collaborative care model, can provide integrated health and behavioral health care. The authors pointed to 70 randomized controlled trials showing that the collaborative care approach to treating depression produced more cost-effective services as well as better patient outcomes than the usual care across diverse practice settings and patient populations. Traditional fee-for-service reimbursement programs have brought about barriers to the widespread implementation of collaborative care, but new reimbursement models using capitated, case-rate payments, or pay-for-performance mechanisms might provide new collaborative care opportunities. Collaborative care in Medicaid, and in integrated care programs for patients with dual eligibility for Medicare and Medicaid, could substantially improve medical and mental health outcomes and functioning, as well as reduce health care costs (Unutzer et al., 2013).

The Integrated Behavioral Health Project in California identified additional positive clinical outcomes to integrated care, including mental health, SUDs, and physical health issues as identified here:

Effects on depression:
- A study on the efficacy of collaborative chronic care models for mental health disorders found significant positive effects across disorders and care settings for depression, physical quality of life, and social functioning. Seventy-eight articles were reviewed (Woltmann et al., 2012).
- Strengthening depression management in primary care settings on an ongoing basis resulted in improved long-term treatment effectiveness, increasing the number of days free of depression impairment for 2 years compared to the usual care, 648 days versus 568 days (Rost, Pyne, Dickinson, & LoSassco, 2005).
- Older African American and Latino primary care clients assigned to an integrated intervention had lower depression severity and less health-related functional impairment than usual care participants (64% vs. 95%) at 12 months (Arean et al., 2005).
- Complex interventions that incorporated clinical education, an enhanced role of the nurse (nurse case manager), a greater intervention between primary and secondary care (consultation-liaison), and telephone medication consultation delivered by practical nurses or trained counselors were effective strategies for improving client outcomes for depression in primary care settings. These findings were based on an analysis of 36 studies (Gilbody, Whitty, Grimshaw, & Thomas, 2003). In a second article by the same authors, 12,555 clients in 37 randomized studies found that depression outcomes were significantly better at 6 months as compared with usual treatment. This outcome was directly related to medication compliance and the professional background and method of supervision of the case managers (Gilbody, Bower, Fletcher, Richards, & Sutton, 2006).
- Veterans with depression randomly assigned to collaborative care experienced an average of 14.6 more days free of depression than veterans receiving usual care, over a 9-month period (Liu et al., 2003).
- Clients scoring high on depression assigned to stepped care intervention (including client education, adjustment of pharmacotherapy and

proactive outcome monitoring) experienced less interference in their family, work, and social activities than clients receiving usual primary care. This study involved a randomized controlled trial of four primary care HMO clinics (Lin et al., 2000).

Effects on panic disorder and bipolar disorder:

- Primary care clients with panic disorders randomly assigned to a collaborative care intervention (systematic patient education and approximately two visits with an on-site consulting psychiatrist) experienced an average of 74.2 more days free of anxiety during the 12-month intervention compared to clients receiving the usual primary care (Katon, Roy-Byrne, Russo, & Cowley, 2002).
- Clients treated for bipolar disorders were randomly assigned to usual care or usual care plus a systematic care management program (initial assessment and care planning, monthly telephone monitoring including brief symptom assessment and medication monitoring, feedback to and coordination with the mental health treatment team, and a structured group psychoeducational program, all provided by a nurse care manager). The clients who received the added systematic care management program had lower mean ratings of mania over a 12-month follow-up period and about one third less time in hypomanic or manic episodes (2.6 weeks vs. 1.7 weeks; Simon et al., 2005).

Effects on drug abuse:

- Adult drug abusers who met with an addiction peer counselor just once during a routine physician visit and received a follow-up booster phone call were less likely to continue drug use than clients who were randomly assigned usual care. Among cocaine users, 22.3% reported abstinence 6 months after enrollment compared to 16.9% of the control group. Among heroin users, the results were 40.2% compared to 30.6% (Bernstein & Bernstein, 2005).
- The potentially important role of medical care and the integration of substance abuse treatment with primary care is supported by a study of 598 chemical dependency clients who were in remission after 5 years as a result of higher primary care engagement (Mertens, Flisher, Satre, & Weisner, 2008).

Effects on physical health:

- Clients with serious mental illnesses receiving care in VA mental health programs with colocated general medical clinics were more likely to receive adequate medical care than clients in programs without colocated clinics based on a nationally representative sample (Kilbourne et al., 2011).
- Clients with serious mental illnesses receiving services in a mental health center who were randomly assigned to medical care management (care mangers who provided communication and advocacy with medical providers as well as health education and assistance in overcoming harriers

to health care) received higher levels of preventive and cardiometabolic services. They also scored higher on mental health screenings compared to the usual treatment group (Druss et al., 2010).

Table 4 provides an extensive list of model integrated mental health and SUD services with quality outcomes, health care costs, (when available) and key model components. Table 4 includes 18 model integration projects and activities. These models include a randomly assigned experimental design study, nonprofit managed care plan, health insurer, medical clinic and VA clinic, African-American-focused evaluation study, Chronic Disease Self-Management Program study, and cost studies. Some of the projects are focused only on mental health issues, but others include SUDs. One model, Puentes Integrated Medical Care, includes a medical home for people with a history of injection drug use or homelessness.

## ECONOMIC BENEFITS OF INTEGRATED CARE: THE BUSINESS CASE

Controlling health care costs while improving clinical outcomes remains a primary reason Congress passed the ACA legislation. The current financial and human costs of our health care system are enormous. According to Manderscheid (2010), the "national disease care system" in the United States cost $2.6 trillion in 2010, $2.5 trillion of which was for disease treatment ($2.0 trillion was for chronic illness treatment). Mauer and Jarvis (2010) pointed out that the "business case" for integrated care is supported by the substantially higher health care costs without integration. For example:

- Depression is ranked seventh as a cause of increasing medical costs in a national survey of employers. It is the greatest cause of lost productivity among workers. People with depression have an annual health care cost of $6,000 per year, twice the cost compared to those without depression.
- 49% of Medicaid beneficiaries with disabilities have a psychiatric illness, and 52% of those who have both Medicare and Medicaid have a psychiatric illness.
- $5.4 million in health care savings could be achieved for each group of 100,000 insured members with only a 10% reduction in the excess health care costs of patients with cooccurring psychiatric disorders through an effective integrated care program.

The authors further suggested that the business case for integrated care is supported by the following:

- Improved health of the population.

- Studies show that treatment protocols, including integrated care, for people with Type 2 diabetes and depression have twice the effectiveness in depression care, resulting in improved physical functioning and decreased pain.
- Case management focused on the health status of people with serious mental illness significantly improved the risk scores for cardiovascular disease.
- Improving the health of those with SUDs might benefit the health of their families as well, according to a Kaiser Northern California study. When the family member with an addiction was abstinent for at least 1 year after treatment, the health care costs for the family were reduced to the level of the control group.
- Enhance the patient experience of care (including quality, access, and reliability).
  - Individuals with serious mental illnesses have a 53% greater chance of being hospitalized for diabetes that could have been managed in an outpatient setting.
  - Adding attention to the health care needs of individuals served in a mental health setting resulted in improved access to routine preventive services, such as immunizations, hypertension screening, and cholesterol screening.
- Reduce, or at least control, the per capita cost of total health care.
  - Studies show that mental health and SUD treatment improve health status and reduce total health care costs. For example, depression care management for Medicaid enrollees can reduce overall health care costs by $2,040 per year per enrollee with reductions in emergency department visits and hospital days.
  - A Kaiser Northern California study showed that persons who received SUD treatment had a 35% reduction in inpatient cost, 39% reduction in emergency room cost, and a 26% reduction in total medical cost, compared with a matched control group.

Further evidence of cost savings, as well as increased productive capacity, that supports the business case for integrated care, includes the following:

- The economic benefits of integrated care include doubling the success rate for depression treatment in primary care settings at a cost of only $264 per case. The result is a positive cost-effectiveness index of $491 per case of depression treated.
- Meta-analysis of 57 controlled studies showed a net 27% cost savings with integrated services.
- There is a 40% savings in the cost of Medicaid patients receiving targeted behavioral health treatment.

## THE AFFORDABLE CARE ACT AND INTEGRATED BEHAVIORAL HEALTH CARE

**TABLE 4** Models of Integrated Mental Health and Substance Use Services That Improve Quality Outcomes and Lower Health Care Costs

| Impact mental health projects | |
|---|---|
| **1. IMPACT research trials** | |
| Brief description | • 1,801 depressed older adults in primary care randomly assigned to IMPACT care or usual care |
| | • 18 primary care clinics |
| | • 8 health care organizations in 5 states |
| | • 8 diverse health care systems |
| | • 450 primary care physicians |
| Quality outcomes | • Greater satisfaction with depression care |
| | • Initial treatments are rarely sufficient—several changes in treatment are often necessary (stepped care) |
| | • Doubled effectiveness of care for depression (50% improvement at 12 months) |
| | • Effective for Black and Latino populations |
| | • Improved physical functioning (SF-12 Physical Function Component Summary Score) |
| | • As depression improves, so does pain |
| Health care costs | • Lowers long-term (4-year) health care costs—$3,363 less total cost over 4 years, including cost of IMPACT intervention |
| | • Intervention patients had lower health care costs in every cost category (outpatient and inpatient mental health specialty costs, outpatient and inpatient medical and surgical costs, pharmacy costs, and other outpatient costs) |
| Key model components | • Screening and systematic outcomes tracking (e.g., PHQ-9) to know when change in treatment is needed |
| | • Active care management to facilitate changes in medication, behavioral activation |
| | • Consultation with mental health specialist if patients not improving |
| **2. DIAMOND/Adaptation of IMPACT model** | |
| Brief description | • Integrated adult depression care management supported by 8 commercial payors and state Medicaid plan in Minnesota. |
| | • Organized by the Institute of Clinical Systems Improvement (ICSI) |
| | • Evidence-based depression care management available in ∼90 primary care clinics statewide (from small practices to the Mayo Clinic) |
| Quality outcomes | • Initial findings for those in the program at least 6 months show 42% in remission and an additional 12% with at least a 50% improvement in their depression scores |
| Health care Costs | • No data yet available—evaluation in process |
| Key model components | • Screening expanded beyond depression to include anxiety/PTSD, bipolar, and substance use screening |
| | • Testing a bundled payment method for every patient being tracked on the project registry Common payment code for IMPACT care covers: Trained care managers (social workers, licensed counselors, nurses); Psychiatric consultation (weekly); PHQ-9 follow-up |
| | • Detailed description of key processes below |
| **3. IMPACT applications to patients with diabetes** | |
| Brief description | • A series of analyses of the IMPACT model specifically in relation to depression in patients with diabetes tested applicability to Latino |

*(Continued)*

# THE AFFORDABLE CARE ACT AND INTEGRATED BEHAVIORAL HEALTH CARE

**TABLE 4** Continued

Impact mental health projects

|  |  |
|---|---|
| | adults, a general population of adults, and older adults in the original IMPACT trials |
| | • Depression is twice as common among people with diabetes as in the general population and is believed to adversely affect the complex self-care activities necessary for diabetes control |
| Quality outcomes | • The combined diabetes and depression care manager tested in the Project Dulce/IMPACT pilot was both feasible and highly effective in reducing depressive symptoms; depression scores declined by an average of 7.5 points from 14.8 to 7.3 |
| | • The Pathways/Group Health Cooperative (GHC) study reported that mean depression scores were significantly lower at 6 and 12 months, and that, over 24 months, patients accumulated a mean of 61 additional days free of depression |
| | • The subanalysis from the IMPACT trials of older adults with diabetes found that the intervention was a high-value investment, associated with high clinical benefits at no greater ambulatory cost than usual care |
| Health care costs | • Depression cooccurring with diabetes is associated with higher health services costs (50–100% higher) |
| | • The Pathways/GHC study reported outpatient health services costs that averaged $314 less than the control group. The estimated cost savings was $300 per patient treated (e.g., an investment of $800 in depression treatment was offset by a decrease of $1,100 in costs of general medical care) |
| | • When an additional day free of depression is valued at $19, the net economic benefit of the Pathways/GHC intervention was $952 per patient treated |
| | • The subanalysis from the IMPACT trials of older adults with diabetes found that the intervention was a high-value investment. In the diabetes subgroup, in the first year, there was a $665 increase in outpatient costs and in the second year, there was a $639 cost savings. Total medical costs, over 2 years, were $869 less in the intervention group |
| Key model components | • Project Dulce/IMPACT project added a bilingual, bicultural depression care manager to an existing diabetes management team |
| | • Clients averaged 6.7 visits with the depression care manager |
| | • Project Dulce included peer-led self-management training |
| | • The Pathways/GHC study had specialized nurses delivering a 12-month stepped-care depression treatment program (initial visit followed by contacts twice a month during acute phase, decreasing depending on clinical response) beginning with either problem-solving treatment psychotherapy or a structured antidepressant pharmacotherapy program; subsequent treatment was adjusted according to clinical response |

Health plan mental health integration projects

|  |  |
|---|---|
| 4. Colorado Access Brief description | • Nonprofit managed care plan with contract as regional Medicaid HMO and Regional MH Carve-Out |
| | • 64% of enrollees in Aged/Blind/Disabled Medicaid aid code |
| | • Part of MacArthur Initiative and RWJ Depression in Primary Care Project |

*(Continued)*

# THE AFFORDABLE CARE ACT AND INTEGRATED BEHAVIORAL HEALTH CARE

**TABLE 4** Continued

| Health plan mental health integration projects | |
|---|---|
| | • Analysis of overlapping populations in two plans showed that 40% of people had a mental health diagnosis, yet only 33% had ever seen a mental health provider, and for most, this was a one-time visit |
| Quality outcomes | • The focus of this analysis was health care cost, data not available on outcomes |
| Health care costs | • Emergency department visits/1,000: From 220.3 at 12 months pre to 163 at 24 months post |
| | • Office visits/1,000: From 211.8 at 12 months pre to 358.2 at 24 months post |
| | • Admits/1,000: From 49.7 at 12 months pre to 37.4 at 24 months post |
| | • Days/1,000: From 232.5 at 12 months pre to 205.4 at 24 months post |
| | • Savings of $170 per month, $2,040 per year |
| | • 12.9% reduction in costs in high-cost, high-risk patients |
| Key model components | • Centralized care management in the plan, with telephonic, on site in primary care or in-community care contacts based on risk stratification |
| | • Care managers were nurses or mental health specialists |
| | • Registry to track PHQ-9, treatment adherence, self-management goals and progress, educational interventions, case management, and comorbid disorders and treatments |
| | • Focus on top 2–3% of population using Kronick risk assessment methods |
| | • Three levels of risk stratification, based on PHQ-9, presence of psychiatric or medical comorbidities, high risk for nonadherence, psychosocial stressors, and treatment-resistant depression |
| 5. Aetna | |
| Brief description | • Integration with primary care providers (PCPs) |
| |   • Depression |
| |   • Pediatrics |
| |   • SBIRT |
| |   • Integrated behavioral health |
| Quality outcomes | • 61% drop in PHQ-9 score between admission and discharge (45% have moderate to severe depression >14 on PHQ-9) |
| | • 48% of enrollees with major depression achieve PHQ-9 < 5 (remission) |
| Health care costs | • Cost impact: reduction on completion ($n = 375$) |
| |   • Emergency department 39% |
| |   • Inpatient 30% |
| |   • Outpatient 47% |
| |   • Psychiatric visit 3% |
| |   • Psychotherapy visits 290% increase |
| | • Net total cost savings 39% |
| Key model components | • Health plan penetration |
| |   • Office identification by volume, diagnosis, and pharmacy claims |
| |   • Creation of virtual disease registry |
| |   • Initiative with employer groups and multiple health plans |
| | • Infrastructure-practice models |
| |   • Quality infrastructure—EMR, registries, population management |

*(Continued)*

# THE AFFORDABLE CARE ACT AND INTEGRATED BEHAVIORAL HEALTH CARE

**TABLE 4** Continued

Health plan mental health integration projects

- Facilitated implementation—PCP office implementation toolkit
- Web site: http://www.aetna.com/ aetnadepressionmanagement/
- Role of office administrator-training module
- Lack of utilization—adoption and persistency
  - Academic detailing
  - Office manager single point of contact
  - Recurrent communication—E-mail reminders
  - Community physician thought leader communications
- Reluctant to refer to health plan care management
  - Focus care management on facilitated access to behavioral health
- Behavioral health provider network issues
  - Conceptual framework and training models
  - Training behavioral health and PCPs
  - Incentives
- Health plan integration
  - Similar to provider integration and cultural issues
  - Integration of behavioral health and medical health data set and care management system
  - Data sharing and privacy issues
- Behavioral health financing
  - Transactional reimbursement and claims payment systems
  - Silos between behavioral health and medical financing—carve in vs. carve out
  - Lack of standardized reimbursement codes to support screening, case management
  - Funding cost of integration

Health care in mental health settings

| | |
|---|---|
| 6. VA integrated care clinic | |
| Brief description | • A medical clinic was established to manage routine medical problems of patients with SMI at a VA mental health clinic |
| | • Study randomized 120 veterans to either the integrated care clinic or usual care, followed for 1 year |
| Quality outcomes | • Significantly increased the rates and number of visits to medical providers, reduced likelihood of emergency room use |
| | • Significantly improved quality of most routine preventive services (15/17) |
| | • Significantly improved scores on SF-36 Health Related Quality of Life |
| Health care costs | • Program cost-neutral from a VA perspective (primary care costs offset by reduction in inpatient costs) |
| Key model components | • Medical clinic colocated in VA specialty mental health clinic |
| | • Nurse practitioner provided the bulk of medical services; a care manager provided patient education and referrals to mental health and medical specialists |
| 7. PCARE (Primary Care Access, Referral, and Evaluation) Study | |
| Brief description | • 400 persons with SMI randomized to either care management or usual care |

(*Continued*)

## TABLE 4 Continued

### Health care in mental health settings

| | |
|---|---|
| Quality outcomes | • Study setting: inner-city, academically affiliated CMHC in Atlanta, GA. Population largely poor, African American, with SMI<br>• Subjects in PCARE received an average of 58.7% of recommended preventive services (compared to a rate of 21.8% in the usual care group)<br>• Subjects in PCARE received a significantly higher proportion of evidence-based services for cardio metabolic conditions (34.9% vs. 27.7%)<br>• Subjects in PCARE were more likely to report having a primary care provider than those in usual care (71.2% vs. 51.9%)<br>• Improved SF-36 scores<br>  • Mental Component Summary Score: 8.0% improvement in intervention versus 1.1% decline in the control group<br>  • Physical Component Summary Score: 1.9% improvement in intervention versus 2.8% decline in control, not statistically significant<br>• Among subjects with fasting blood tests, Framingham risk scores for cardiovascular disease at 12 months were significantly better for PCARE than usual care (6.9% risk vs. 9.8%)<br>  • The intervention group showed an 11.8% improvement at the 1 year evaluation and the control group showed a 19.5% increase in risk, not statistically significant |
| Health care costs | • The focus of this analysis was health care improvement, data not available on costs |
| Key model components | • Two nurse care managers (one psychiatric, one public health) help patients get access to and follow-up with regular medical care, but do not provide any direct medical services<br>• Examples of services include patient education; scheduling appointments, advocacy (e.g., accompanying patients to appointments, communicating with PCPs)<br>  • Role of care manager: primary point of contact, clinician, advocate, liaison, educator, coach/cheerleader, translator |

### 8. HARP (Health and Recovery Peer) Project

| | |
|---|---|
| Brief description | • Adapting Stanford's Chronic Disease Self-Management Program (CDSMP), for mental health consumers<br>• In general populations with chronic illnesses, the CDSMP has been shown to improve self-efficacy and reduce unnecessary health service use<br>• Focus groups used to identify key areas needed to be changed or added<br>• Physical wellness fits naturally into existing peer-based recovery programs and peer workforce |
| Quality outcomes | • At 6 months, patient activation clinically and statistically significantly higher in HARP group than control, in addition:<br>  • Additional 40 minutes per week in moderate to vigorous exercise<br>  • 14.2% improvement in medication adherence compared to 7.3% decline in control<br>  • 16.3% increase in improvement on the Health Related Quality of Life Physical Component Summary compared to 8.1% in control |
| Health care costs | • The focus of this analysis was health care improvement; data were not available on costs |

## THE AFFORDABLE CARE ACT AND INTEGRATED BEHAVIORAL HEALTH CARE

**TABLE 4** Continued

| Health care in mental health settings | |
| --- | --- |
| Key model components | • The CDSMP is a peer-led, annualized program designed to improve individuals' self-management of chronic illnesses<br>• Set short- and long-term goals, identify the specific steps and actions to be taken to pursue those goals<br>• Rank confidence, on a scale of 1–10, in achieving these objectives; if the confidence is less than 7, reexamine the barriers<br>• Six-session format focuses on promoting self-efficacy through goal setting and action plans<br>• Sessions focus on health and nutrition, exercise, and being a more effective patient<br>• Changes to CDSMP<br>  • Addition of content on mental health and general health interaction symptoms and systems was added<br>  • Mental health certified peer leaders trained to become master CDSMP trainers<br>  • Diet and exercise recommendations tailored for socioeconomic status of public sector population<br>• Socioeconomic status issues are critical to consider in developing programs in this population<br>• Poverty is likely a major cause of excess morbidity and mortality in persons with SMI; influences everything from diet and exercise to access to medical care in this population |

| Northern California Kaiser Permanente substance use studies | |
| --- | --- |
| **9. Integrated Medical Care** | |
| Brief description | • Internally operated adult outpatient and day treatment substance use program with integrated primary care (control group had independent primary care)<br>• 1.25 full-time equivalent (FTE) PCPs with training in substance use, 1 FTE medical assistant, and 1.8 FTE nurses served the 318 patients assigned to integrated care<br>• Focus on individuals with substance abuse-related medical conditions (SAMCs) |
| Quality outcomes | • Significantly higher abstinence rates compared to SAMC independent care patients<br>• Significantly reduced inpatient rates compared to SAMC independent care patients<br>• Significantly more integrated care patients were newly diagnosed with SAMC conditions |
| Health care costs | • For SAMC integrated care patients, average medical costs (excluding addiction treatment) decreased from $470.39 PMPM to $226.86 PMPM |
| Key model components | • Traditional substance use outpatient and day treatment, group based, with 10 months of aftercare<br>• Modalities included supportive group therapy, education, relapse prevention, family-oriented therapy, 12-step meetings, and individual counseling as needed<br>• Combined with standard PCP practice team with MDs, nurses, and MA |

*(Continued)*

# THE AFFORDABLE CARE ACT AND INTEGRATED BEHAVIORAL HEALTH CARE

**TABLE 4** Continued

Northern California Kaiser Permanente substance use studies

**10. Pre/post substance use treatment and medical costs**

| | |
|---|---|
| Brief description | • Analysis of average medical cost PMPM in 18 months pre- and post-substance use treatment using historical data |
| Quality outcomes | • The focus of this analysis was health care costs; data were not available on outcomes |
| Health care costs | • Substance use treatment group had a 35% reduction in inpatient cost, 39% reduction in emergency room cost, and a 26% reduction in total medical cost, compared with matched control group |
| Key model components | • Not specified, assume traditional substance use outpatient and day treatment |

**11. The role of psychiatry in 5-year outcomes**

| | |
|---|---|
| Brief description | • Analysis of psychiatric services for adults with psychiatric symptoms after substance use treatment using historical data |
| | • Comparison of abstinence at 5 years after treatment for those who subsequently received 2.1 or more hours of psychiatric services per year compared to those with less or no psychiatric services |
| Quality outcomes | • Those who received 2.1 or more hours of psychiatric services per year were 2.22 times more likely to be abstinent at 5 years after substance use treatment |
| Health care costs | • Those with high psychiatric severity at initiation of treatment had $1,000 PMPM, reduced to about $300 PMPM at 5 years |
| Key model components | • Provision of psychiatric services for individuals with psychiatric symptoms after substance use treatment, with 2.1 hours or more per year demonstrating contribution to abstinence |

**12. Role of primary care in 5-year outcomes**

| | |
|---|---|
| Brief description | • Analysis of continuing care and effect on remission, using historical data |
| | • Continuing care defined as: |
| |   • Substance use treatment when needed |
| |   • Psychiatric services when needed |
| |   • Primary care at least every year |
| Quality outcomes | • Patients receiving continuing care were more than twice as likely to be remitted at each follow-up over 9 years |
| | • Those receiving continuing care in the prior interval were less likely to have emergency room visits and hospitalizations subsequently (even if not in remission) |
| Health care costs | • Continuing care reduced inappropriate utilization even when not in remission |
| Key model components | • Continuing care defined as: |
| |   • Substance use treatment when needed |
| |   • Psychiatric services when needed |
| |   • Primary care at least every year |

**13. Costs of family members**

| | |
|---|---|
| Brief description | • Analysis of the medical conditions and costs of family members of individuals with substance use conditions using historical data |
| Quality outcomes | • The focus of this analysis was health care costs; data were not available on outcomes |
| Health care costs | • Pretreatment, families of all substance use patients have higher medical costs than control families |
| | • Adult family members have significantly higher prevalence of 12 medical conditions compared with control group; child family |

*(Continued)*

# THE AFFORDABLE CARE ACT AND INTEGRATED BEHAVIORAL HEALTH CARE

**TABLE 4** Continued

### Northern California Kaiser Permanente substance use studies

|  |  |
|---|---|
|  | members have significantly higher prevalence of 9 medical conditions |
|  | • At 2 to 5 years postintake for substance use services, if family member with substance use condition were abstinent at 1 year, family members had similar average PMPM medical costs as control group |
|  | • Family members of substance use patients who were not abstinent at 1 year had a trajectory of increasing medical cost relative to control group |
| Key model components | • Not specified, assume traditional substance use outpatient and day treatment |

### Other substance use studies

**14. U.S. Preventive Services Task Force (USPSTF)**

| Brief description | • A ranking of 25 preventive services recommended by the USPSTF based on clinically preventable burden and cost effectiveness |
|---|---|
| Quality outcomes | • Primary care-based counseling interventions for risky/harmful alcohol use found that good-quality brief multicontact counseling interventions (defined as an initial session up to 15 minutes long, plus follow-up contacts) reduced risky and harmful alcohol use |
|  | • Alcohol screening and intervention rated at the same level as such established practices as colorectal cancer screening and treatment and hypertension screening and treatment in clinically preventable burden and cost effectiveness |
| Health care costs | • Findings suggest that investments in regular screening are likely to be very cost effective from the health-system perspective and to be cost saving from the societal perspective |
| Key model components | • Primary care-based counseling interventions for risky/harmful alcohol use with good-quality brief multicontact counseling interventions (defined as an initial session up to 15 minutes long, plus follow-up contacts) |
|  | • Effective interventions include advice, feedback, goal setting, and additional contacts for further assistance and support |

Support such as:
- Commitment to planning
- Allocation of resources and staff to consistently identify risk/harmful alcohol-using patients
- Delivery resources such as clinician training, prompts, materials, reminders, and referral resources

**15. Screening and Brief Intervention (SBI) studies**

| Brief description | • An overview of the effectiveness of SBI as a comprehensive, integrated, public health approach |
|---|---|
| Quality outcomes | • Trauma patients: 48% fewer reinjury at 18-month follow-up, 50% less likely to rehospitalize |
|  | • ED screening: reduced UI arrests |
|  | • Physician offices: 20% fewer motor vehicle crashes over 48-month follow-up |
| Health care costs | • Randomized trial in United Kingdom: $2.30 cost savings for each $1.00 spent in intervention |
|  | • Randomized trial at U.S. Level 1 trauma center: $3.81 cost savings for each $1.00 spent in intervention |

*(Continued)*

# THE AFFORDABLE CARE ACT AND INTEGRATED BEHAVIORAL HEALTH CARE

**TABLE 4** Continued

Other substance use studies

| | |
|---|---|
| Key model components | • Randomized trial in primary care clinic: $4.30 cost savings for each $1.00 spent in intervention<br>• Screening: Very brief screening that identifies substance-related problems<br>• Brief intervention: Raises awareness of risks and motivates client toward acknowledgment of problem<br>• Brief treatment: Cognitive behavioral work with clients who acknowledge risks and are seeking help<br>• Referral: Referral of those with more serious addictions |

16. Washington State substance use and medical cost studies

| | |
|---|---|
| Brief description | • Analyses of Medicaid medical expenses prior to specialty substance use treatment and over a 5-year follow-up were compared to Medicaid expenses for the untreated population |
| Quality outcomes | • The focus of these analyses was health care costs; data were not available on outcomes |
| Health care costs | • For the Supplemental Security Income (SSI) population, average monthly medical costs were $414 per month higher for those not receiving treatment, and with the cost of the treatment added in, there was still a net cost offset of $252 per month or $3,024 per year<br>• The net cost offset rose to $363 per month for those who completed treatment<br>• For SSI recipients with opiate addiction, cost offsets rose to $899 per month for those who remain in methadone treatment for at least 1 year<br>• In the SSI population, average monthly emergency department costs were lower for those treated—the number of visits per year was 19% lower and the average cost per visit was 29% lower, almost offsetting the average monthly cost of treatment<br>• For frequent emergency department users (12 or more visits per year) there was a 17% reduction in average visits for those who entered, but didn't complete substance use treatment and a 48% reduction for those who did complete treatment |
| Key model components | • Details of substance use treatments not discussed in detail, but likely included full range including residential, intensive outpatient, outpatient, and methadone maintenance |

17. Puentes Integrated Medical Care

| | |
|---|---|
| Brief description | • Primary care clinic colocated with an outpatient methadone clinic, targeted to individuals with history of injection drug use and the homeless population; located within a large county health care system, Santa Clara Valley Health and Hospital System (CA) |
| Quality outcomes | • Primary care visits increased from 2.8 visits to 5.9 visits in the same time frames<br>• More than half of patients who began care at Puentes still use care 5 years later, suggesting this is a medical home for them |
| Health care costs | • Emergency room and urgent care visits decreased from 3.8 visits in the 18 months prior to the clinic opening to 0.8 visits in the first 18 months of clinic opening |
| Key model components | • A medical home for individuals with a history of injection drug use or homelessness<br>• Includes traditional medical care, hepatitis C treatment, psychology and psychiatry services, and a pain clinic; integrated treatment team composed of professionals with distinct areas of expertise who work together to treat the whole patient (fostered by single, |

*(Continued)*

# THE AFFORDABLE CARE ACT AND INTEGRATED BEHAVIORAL HEALTH CARE

**TABLE 4** Continued

Other substance use studies

|  |  |
|---|---|
|  | shared office space and formal case conferences) |
|  | • Outreach meets patients where they are and build trust through mobile services |
|  | • Open access and "chat room" with facilitated dialogue while waiting to be seen |
|  | • Specialty groups for patients with specific medical conditions |

18. Downtown Emergency Service Center (DESC) 1811 Program

|  |  |
|---|---|
| Brief description | • Seattle Housing First model targeted to serve homeless individuals with severe substance use or cooccurring conditions; health and mental health/substance use staff was wrapped around the housing through DESC's capacities as a mental health/substance use provider and with a primary care clinic focused on the homeless population |
| Quality outcomes | • Alcohol use by Housing First participants decreased by about one third |
| Health care costs | • The program saved more than $4 million over the first year of operation; a significant portion of the cost offsets were caused by decreases in residents' use of Medicaid-funded health services |
| Key model components | • Housing First model targeted to serve homeless individuals with severe substance use or cooccurring conditions; health and mental health/substance use staff were wrapped around the housing |

*Note.* EBP = evidence-based practice; SMI = serious mental illness; MA = medical assistant. *Source*: Mauer and Jarvis (2010).

- There is up to 70% savings in in-patient costs with integrated care in older patients.
- Integrated care services produced an average of 20% to 30% overall cost savings in the studies reviewed.
- Estimates of the revenue ceiling of a health care system are closely tied to the productive capacity of the medical providers.
- Current capacity in primary care settings is limited due to frequent management of behavioral health conditions: 50% of medical practice time is directed toward behavioral health conditions.
- Integrated behavioral health services "leverage" behavioral health patients out of primary care physician practice schedules. Primary care physicians have more time to see medical patients with higher priority needs (Bureau of Primary Health Care, n.d.).

## BARRIERS TO INTEGRATION

The AHRQ (2012) identified barriers to integration as:

- Workforce issues, such as the differences in workplace cultures for behavioral health versus primary care staff.

- Financial barriers, including:
  - The need for separate billing codes for each intervention by a team member.
  - State Medicaid limitations on payments for same-day billing for a physical health and a mental health service.
  - Lack of reimbursement for collaborative care and care management related to mental health services.
  - Medicaid disallowance of reimbursement when primary care practitioners submit bills listing only a mental health diagnosis.

Table 5 lists financial and organizational barriers to integration with strategies to address the barriers. One issue Table 5 does not include is the need for comprehensive, integrated care systems to fully integrate their electronic health record (EHR) technology. A fully integrated EHR system is necessary

**TABLE 5** Barriers to Integrating Primary Care and Mental Health Care

| Type of barrier | Strategy |
| --- | --- |
| Financial<br>• Carved out mental health services<br>• Consultation between providers not compensated<br>• Care manager not always eligible for compensation<br>• No reimbursement for two encounters on same day with different professionals (public funding)<br>• Mental health services carved out of general medical services<br>• No reimbursement for telephone consultation | • Permitting credentialed primary care physicians (PCPs) to bill carve out managed behavioral health care organization for mental health care<br>• Allow PCPs to bill for behavioral health visit, even when it occurs simultaneously with general medical care visit<br>• Care manager employed or under contract with health plan<br>• Intervention paid through quality improvement funding<br>• Care managers (behavioral health specialists) employed by health organization<br>• Care specialists "loaned" to primary care, but billed to payer from specialty sector<br>• Negotiated pricing for care management services<br>• Creation of new CPT codes for billing care management services<br>• Pay for performance funds |
| Organizational<br>• Resistance to change<br>• Staffing: Availability of mental health specialists, acceptance of new roles<br>• Time: Balancing competing demands and burden of case identification<br>• Expertise and comfort dealing with mental health problems<br>• Privacy concerns: HIPAA | • Identification of leaders to support and promote the integration<br>• Training of allied professionals (physician extenders) to provide mental health services and care management<br>• Provider education and support<br>• Telemedicine |

*Note.* CPT = current procedural terminology. *Source*: Butler et al. (2008).

for billing under ACA, managing clinical care, collecting patient data, and making integrated care possible. However, EHR systems are costly due to the Health Insurance Portability and Accountability Act (HIPAA) requirements. Conversion to a fully integrated system is very labor intensive and creates a barrier, especially for service providers who are already busy with their clinical duties.

DeGruy and Miller at the Department of Family Medicine, University of Colorado School of Medicine, have been working on a primary care and mental health integration project for many years. They seek to not only develop ways for primary care and mental health treatment services to be fully integrated, but to also find ways to achieve financial sustainability for programs at the local level. Nichols, Weinberg, and Barnes (2009) also conducted a community-wide analysis of Grand Junction, CO, in terms of how this city integrated its health and behavioral health services. They found that at the time of the study, the financial resources were not available to sustain a fully integrated system of care. However, with the implementation of ACA and the extensive collaborative work of the local service providers, integrating their system of care might be possible in the near future. The authors offer these lessons applicable to integrated services and the ACA:

- Lesson 1: Vision and incentives are essential to an operational sense of community.
- Lesson 2: Information systems and data sharing are essential for collaboration and trust.
- Lesson 3: Complementary institutions pursuing their comparative advantages facilitate collaboration.
- Lesson #: Primary care is the core of any high-performance health system.

Van Egeren and Huber (n.d.) suggested that additional barriers exist at a practice level when providing mental health services to primary care patients:

- Competing demands and tasks of primary care providers.
- Limitations of specialty mental health services in primary health settings.
- Patient barriers to providing mental health services, such as stigma.
- Organizational barriers: organizational change, time pressures, and sustainability issues (Dall, 2011, pp. 20–22).

## IMPLICATIONS OF INTEGRATION IN ACA FOR UNDERSERVED POPULATIONS

The ACA will expand health insurance coverage to millions of Americans providing virtually universal coverage, largely due to the Medicaid expansion portion of the program. This expansion will include diverse ethnic minorities and others with limited incomes, as well as individuals with disabilities and preexisting medical and behavioral health conditions. Women will be eligible for specialized services within the 10 essential benefits, which include maternity care and 22 covered preventive services. Examples of these preventive services for pregnant women and those who are not pregnant include breast cancer mammography screening, cervical cancer screening, contraception, domestic and interpersonal violence screening and counseling, gestational diabetes screening, HIV screening, osteoporosis screening, tobacco use screening and interventions, sexually transmitted infection counseling, and well-woman visits (Healthcare.gov, n.d.). The ACA also provides children and adolescents with access to 25 covered preventive services, medical and dental care, and behavioral health services during the period in their lives when these services are most important (Healthcare.gov, n.d.).

All of the ACA services must follow the Department of Health and Human Services Office of Minority Health's standards for Culturally and Linguistically Appropriate Services. This requirement should assure high-quality care that takes into consideration the patient's language and culture in delivering health and behavioral health services. However, developing an adequate workforce of appropriately trained, ethnically diverse, bilingual and culturally competent service providers by the time the ACA is fully implemented will be very challenging.

When in jail or prison, individuals retain eligibility for ACA health insurance. Those without health insurance when entering the jail or a prison system can apply for coverage before they are released from custody to have the health insurance when they reenter their communities. Thus, these individuals returning to the community can obtain the mental health and substance abuse services that can help change their lives and reduce the "revolving door" back to incarceration. For example, Assembly Bill 720, proposed California legislation by Nancy Skinner (D-Berkeley) will help assure that individuals in the county jail system can apply for health insurance (Medicaid) before they are released from county jail (California Legislative Information, 2013).

The integrated care provided by the ACA will also help address the stigma of mental illness, SUDs, disabilities, and other medical conditions. Diverse ethnic minority populations experience a disproportionate burden and encounter more personal difficulties caused by stigma, discrimination, and health disparities. For example, due in large part to the effects of stigma, Asian American, Native Hawaiian, and Pacific Islander mental health and SUD patients will tend to seek help first through informal community networks, such as family members, clan, clergy, and alternative health care settings (Chu & Sue, 2011). These patients might also turn to Eastern medical practices, including herbal medicines, often before seeking help at a Western-style health care provider. Some cultures, such as Hmong, might seek the aid of shamans in combination with other forms of care (Fadiman, 1997). Some of these patients interpret their behavioral health symptoms as a spiritual matter or a form of physical illness (U.S. Surgeon General, 2001).

The President's New Freedom Commission on Mental Health (2002) identified the stigma regarding mental illness as one of three major obstacles preventing Americans from seeking care. Ample evidence demonstrates that providing behavioral health services within integrated care settings will reduce their stigma. For example, the World Health Organization (WHO) states that the rationale for integrating mental health services into primary health care is to reduce stigma. This reduces stigma because primary health care services are not necessarily associated with a specific health condition, such as mental illness. As a result, seeking mental health care from a primary health provider, compared to a mental health specialty program, makes the process of seeking care more acceptable to most individuals (and families) and therefore more accessible (WHO, 2007). The ACA will also make appropriate health care available to many more individuals and families who did not previously have the resources to get the care they needed, especially in the early stages of mental illness or an SUD when the chances of recovery are usually better. As more individuals receive the preventive care needed for mental illness and SUDs through the ACA, the effectiveness of treatment in the early stages, increased rate of recovery, and the holistic, integrated care provided by an interdisciplinary team might ameliorate the stigma attached to these diseases.

SAMHSA also supports the rationale that integrated care helps reduce stigma, citing programs such as the PeaceHealth's integration of behavioral health services and primary health care (Brunelle & Porter, 2013). SAMHSA supports the Resource Center to Promote Acceptance, Dignity and Social Inclusion Associated with Mental Health (ADS Center). The purpose of the ADS Center includes addressing mental illness and SUDs in terms of reducing stigma and discrimination (SAMHSA–ADS Center, 2013). The White House National Conference on Mental Health held on June 3, 2013, addressed the stigma of mental illness and announced a national dialogue to encourage people with mental health and substance use issues to seek care. President Barack Obama said, "We know that treatment works and that recovery is fully possible. There should be no difference between seeking care for a broken arm and seeking care for depression." Almost 25% of Americans struggle with mental health or SUDs annually. However, only 40% of people with mental illness and only 10% of people with substance abuse conditions receive any care (Manderscheid, 2013). Hopefully, the integrated care provided by the ACA will reduce stigma and help increase the number of people receiving care for mental illness and SUDs through expanded access to culturally competent behavioral health services. One encouraging development is that some funders are committed to the goals and provisions of the ACA and wish to help make it successful.

An example of such a funder is the California Endowment, which has committed $225 million over 4 years to support the successful implementation of the ACA in California. Dr. Robert Ross, CEO of the foundation said, "We have a golden opportunity to create a health care system that is more accessible, more cost-effective and more prevention-oriented. ...We offer this commitment in a sense of partnership, with humility about the task before us, but with urgency about the opportunity in front of us" (The California Endowment, 2013, p. 1). The funding will support four key initiatives:

- Efforts by the state to jump-start community outreach and enrollment in Medi-Cal and other insurance plans in 2014.
- Expansion of the primary care health workforce in anticipation of increased demand for services for thousands of newly insured Californians.
- Reform the delivery of care to control health care costs through improved management of chronic disease, more care coordination and team-based care.
- Explore public and private avenues to provide more consistent care for the undocumented population of Californians who are excluded from coverage under the ACA.

## CONCLUSION

This discussion regarding the ACA and its provisions for integrated care of health care and behavioral health services revealed many complex issues. For instance, historically, the federal government made various attempts to improve the quality of health services, and reduce fragmentation and costs through services integration. Although these efforts were not always successful, they were instructive. Health care costs are still a major driving force for ACA and its nearly universal health insurance coverage. As all of the provisions are implemented at the state and federal levels, the ACA with its integrated care approach will help reduce costs, improve the quality of care, and reduce the stigma of mental illness, SUDs, disability, and other sensitive health issues.

The ACA faces significant challenges as it addresses full implementation, including complex financing issues with a myriad of public and private health care and behavioral health providers, private insurers, nonprofit and for-profit hospitals, clinics and health plans, and accountable care organizations, to name a few. Additionally, how will the needed workforce be recruited to provide preventive, treatment, and recovery services for the anticipated 32 million newly insured Americans? Funders, such as the California Endowment, might help answer these critical questions as the timetable for full ACA implementation draws near. Clearly, the political will was there to enact the ACA in 2010, but it has been and continues to be a hotly debated political issue. Regardless, it is the most important new public health program in nearly 50 years and a tremendous opportunity for the United States to join the rest of the industrialized world regarding health care benefits. Let us hope that the ACA and its supporters will deliver on the promise to improve the health status of the whole community and make high-quality, affordable health care a right for all Americans.

## REFERENCES

Agency for Healthcare Research and Quality. (2012, January). *Research Activities Newsletter, 377*. Retrieved from http://www.ahrq.gov/news/newsletters/research-activities/jan12/0112RA.pdf

American Psychological Association. (2008). *Presidential Task Force on Integrated Health Care for and Aging Population. Blueprint for change: Achieving integrated health care for an aging population.* Washington, DC: American Psychological Association. Retrieved from https://www.apa.org/pi/aging/programs/integrated/integrated-healthcare-report.pdf

Arean, P., Ayalon, L., Hunkeler, E., Lin, E. H., Tang, L., Harpole, L., ... IMPACT Investigators. (2005). Improving depression care for older, minority patients in primary care. *Medical Care, 43*, 381–390.

Bernstein, J., & Bernstein, E. (2005). Brief encounters can provide motivation to reduce or stop drug abuse. *Drug and Alcohol Dependence, 77*, 49–59.

Blount, A. (2003). Integrated primary care: Organizing the evidence. *Families, Systems, & Health, 21*(2), 121–33.

Boon, H., Mior, S., Barnsley, J., Ashbury, F., & Haig, R. (2009). The difference between integration and collaboration in patient care: Results from key informant interviews working in multiprofessional health care teams. *Journal of Manipulative & Physiological Therapeutics, 32*, 715–722. doi:10.1016/j.jmpt.2009.10.005

Bower P, Gilbody S, Richards, D., et al. (2006, December). Collaborative care for depression in primary care. Making sense of a complex intervention: systematic review and metaregression. *British Journal of Psychiatry, 189*, 484–93.

Brunelle, J., & Porter, R. (2013). *Integrating care helps reduce stigma.* Retrieved from http://www.integration.samhsa.gov/newzs/Integrating_Care_Helps_Reduce_Stigma.pdf

Bureau of Primary Health Care. (n.d.). *Integrating primary care and behavioral health services: A compass and a horizon.* Retrieved from http://www.apa.org/practice/programs/rural/integrating-primary-behavioral.pdf

Butler, M., Kane, R., McAlpine, D., Kathol, R., Fu, S., Hagedorn, H., & Wilt, T. (2008, October). *Integraton of mental health/substance abuse and primary care* (AHRQ Pub. No. 09-E003). Rockville, MD: Agency for Healthcare Research and Quality. Retrieved from http://www.ahrq.gov/research/findings/evidence-based-reports/mhsapc-evidence-report.pdf

Byrd, M. R., O'Donohue, W. T., & Cummings, N. A. (2005). *The case for integrated care: Coordinating behavioral health care with primary care medicine.* In W. T. O'Donohue, M. R. Byrd, N. A. Cummings, et al. (Eds), *Behavioral Integrative*

*Care. Treatments that work in the primary care setting.* New York, NY: Brunner-Routledge.

The California Endowment. (2013, January 17). *The California Endowment's Board of Directors announces commitment of $225 million to support implementation of the Affordable Care Act in California.* Retrieved from http://tcenews.calendow.org/releases/the-california-endowments-board-of-directors-announces-commitment-of-225-million-to-support-implementation-of-the-affordable-care-act-in-california

California Legislative Information. (2013). *AB-720 inmates: Health care enrollment.* Retrieved from http://leginfo.legislature.ca.gov/faces/billNavClient.xhtml?bill_id=201320140AB720

Chu, J. P., & Sue, S. (2011). Asian American mental health: What we know and what we don't know. *Online Readings in Psychology and Culture, 3*(1). Retrieved from http://dx.doi.org/10.9707/2307-0919.1026

Collins, C., Levis Hewson, D., Munger, R., & Wadem, T. (2010). *Evolving models of behavioral health integration in primary care: The Milbank Memorial Fund.* Retrieved from http://www.milbank.org/uploads/documents/10430Evolving-Care/EvolvingCare.pdf

Croghan, T., & Brown, J. (2010, June). *Integrating mental health treatment into the patient centered medical home* (AHRQ Pub. No. 10-0084-EF). Rockville, MD: Agency for Healthcare Research and Quality.

Dall, A. (2011). *Integrated primary care and behavioral health services: Can the model succeed?* San Diego, CA: AGD Consulting. Retrieved from http://www.ibhp.org/uploads/file/lit%20review%20integrated%20care%20final.pdf

Druss, B., von Esenwein, S., Compton, M., Rask, K., Zhao, L., & Parker, R. (2010). A randomized trial of medical care management for community mental health settings: The Primary Care Access, Referral, and Evaluation (PCARE) study. *American Journal of Psychiatry, 167,* 151–159.

Eagleville Hospital. (n.d.). About us. Retrieved from www.eaglevillehospital.org/aboutus.html

Fadiman, A. (1997). *The spirit catches you and you fall down.* New York, NY: Farrar, Straus & Giroux.

Gagne, M. (2005 June). *What is collaborative mental health care? An introduction to the collaborative mental health care framework.* Canadian Collaborative Mental Health Initiative. Available at: http://www.ccmhi.ca/en/products/documents/02-Framework-EN.pdf.

Gilbody, S., Bower, P., Fletcher, J., Richards, D., & Sutton, A. J. (2006). Collaborative care for depression: A cumulative meta-analysis and review of longer-term outcomes. *Archives of Internal Medicine, 166,* 2314–2321.

Gilbody, S., Whitty, P., Grimshaw, J., & Thomas, R. (2003). Educational and organizational interventions to improve the management of depression in primary care: A systematic review. *Journal of the American Medical Association, 289,* 3145–3151.

Healthcare.gov. (n.d.). *What are my preventive care benefits?* Retrieved from https://www.healthcare.gov/what-are-my-preventive-care-benefits/

Heath, B., Wise Romero, P., & Reynolds, K. (2013). *Six levels of collaboration/integration (core descriptions).* Retrieved from http://www.integration.samhsa.gov/integrated-care-models/CIHS_Framework_Final_charts.pdf

Hogg Foundation for Mental Health. (n.d.). The University of Texas at Austin. Available at: http://www.hogg.utexas.edu/programs_ihc.html

Institute of Medicine. (2006). *Improving the quality of health care for mental and substance-use conditions*. Washington, DC: The National Academies Press.

Institute of Medicine Board on Health Care Services. (1981). *Health care in a context of civil rights*. Washington, DC: National Academy Press.

Institute of Medicine Board on Health Care Services. (1982). *Volume 1: Report of a study: Health services integration: Lessons for the 1980s*. Washington, DC: National Academy Press.

Katon, W., Roy-Byrne, P., Russo, J., & Cowley, D. (2002). Cost-effectiveness and cost offset of a collaborative care intervention for primary care patients with panic disorder. *Archives of General Psychiatry, 59*, 1098–1104.

Kilbourne, A., Pirraglia, P., Lai, Z., Bauer, M., Charns, M., Greenwald, D., ... Yano, E. (2011). Quality of general medical care among patients with serious mental illness: Does colocation of services matter? *Psychiatric Services, 62*, 922–928.

Lin, E., VonKorff, M., Russo, J., Katon, W., Simon, G., Unutzer, J., ... Ludman, E. (2000). Can depression treatment in primary care reduce disability? A stepped care approach. *Archives of Family Medicine, 9*, 1052–1058.

Liu, C., Hedrick, S., Chaney, E., Heagerty, P., Felker, B., Hasenberg, N., ... Katon, W. (2003). Cost-effectiveness of collaborative care for depression in a primary care veteran population. *Psychiatric Services, 54*, 698–704.

Manderscheid, R. (2010). *To your health and wealth: Sprinting toward the triple aim*. Washington, DC: National Association of County Behavioral Health and Developmental Disability Directors. Retrieved from http://www.acmha.org/content/summit/2013/Manderscheid_Slides.pdf

Manderscheid, R. (2013). Bringing mental health from the shadows to Main Street America. *Behavioral Healthcare*. Retrieved from http://www.behavioral.net/blogs/ron-manderscheid/bringing-mental-health-shadows-main-street-america

Mauer, B. (2006). *Behavioral health/primary care integration*. Washington, DC: National Council for Community Behavioral Health. Retrieved from http://www.cpca.org/cpca/assets/File/Policy-and-Advocacy/Active-Policy-Issues/MHSA/BehavioralHealthPrimaryCareIntegration-Mauer2006.pdf

Mauer, B., & Jarvis, D. (2010, June 30). *The business case for bidirectional integrated care*. California Integration Policy Initiative. Retrieved from http://old.thenationalcouncil.org/galleries/policy-file/CiMH%20Business%20Case%20for%20Integration%206-30-2010%20Final.pdf

Mertens, J., Flisher, A., Satre, D., & Weisner, C. (2008). The role of medical conditions and primary care services in 5-year substance use outcomes among chemical dependency treatment patients. *Drug and Alcohol Dependency, 98*, 45–53.

National Association of State Mental Health Program Directors. (2005). *Integrating behavioral health and primary care services: Opportunities and challenges for state mental health authorities*. Alexandria, VA: Author. Retrieved from http://www.nasmhpd.org/docs/publications/MDCdocs/Final%20Technical%20Report%200n%20Primary%20Care%20-%20Behavioral%20Health%20Integration.final.pdf

Nichols, L., Weinberg, M., & Barnes, J. (2009). *Grand Junction, Colorado: A health community that works*. Washington, DC: Health Policy Program, New America Foundation. Retrieved from http://newamerica.net/files/inbriefgrandjunction-colorado.pdf

O'Connor, J. (1974). Comprehensive health planning: Dreams and realities. *Milbank Memorial Fund Quarterly, Health and Society, 52*, 391–413. Retrieved from http://www.jstor.org/discover/10.2307/3349510?uid=3739560&uid=2&uid=4&uid=3739256&sid=21102751409487

Office of National Drug Control Policy. (2012). *Fact sheet-screening, brief intervention, and referral to treatment (SBIRT)*. Washington, DC: Author. Retrieved from http://www.whitehouse.gov/sites/default/files/page/files/sbirt_fact_sheet_ondcp-samhsa_7-25-111.pdf

President's New Freedom Commission on Mental Health. (2002). *Achieving the promise: Transforming mental health care in America*. Washington, DC: Author. Retrieved from www.MentalHealthCommission.gov

Rost, K., Pyne, J., Dickinson, L. M., & LoSassco, A. (2005). Cost-effectiveness of enhancing primary care depression management on an ongoing basis. *Annals of Family Medicine, 3*, 7–14.

Robinson, P. J., & Reiter, Jt. (2007). *Behavioral consultation and primary care. A guide to integrating services*. New York, NY: Springer Science.

SAMHSA–HRSA Center for Integrated Health Solutions. (2006). *MH/primary care integration options*. Retrieved from http://www.integration.samhsa.gov/integrated-care-models/Doherty-McDaniel-Baird-Reynolds_MH-PC_Integration_Options.pdf

SAMHSA–HRSA Center for Integrated Health Solutions. (n.d.-a). *About CIHS*. Retrieved from http://www.integration.samhsa.gov/about-us/about-cihs

SAMHSA–HRSA Center for Integrated Health Solutions. (n.d.-b). *Four quadrant model*. Retrieved from http://www.integration.samhsa.gov/clinical-practice/four_quadrant_model.pdf

SAMHSA–HRSA Center for Integrated Health Solutions. (n.d.-c). *What is integrated care?* Retrieved from http://www.integration.samhsa.gov/about-us/what-is-integrated-care

Shortell, S. M., Gillies, R. R., Anderson, D. A., et al. (2000). *Remaking health care in America: Building organized delivery systems*. 2nd ed. San Francisco: Jossey-Bass Publishers.

Simon, G., Ludman, E., Unutzer, J., Bauer, M., Operskalski, B., & Rutter, C. (2005). Randomized trial of a population-based care program for people with bipolar disorder. *Psychological Medicine, 35*, 13–24.

Smith, S. M., Allwright, S., & O'Dowd, T. (2007). Effectiveness of shared care across the interface between primary and specialty care in chronic disease management. *Cochrane Database of Systematic Reviews, (3)*:CD004910.

Stern, J. (2008). *Community health planning*. Falls Church, VA: American Health Planning Association. Retrieved from http://www.ahpanet.org/files/Community_Health_Planning_09.pdf

Substance Abuse and Mental Health Services Administration. (2011). *Leading change: A plan for SAMHSA's roles and actions 2011–2014. Executive summary and introduction* (HHS Pub. No. SMA 11–4629 Summary). Rockville,

MD: Author. Retrieved from http://store.samhsa.gov/shin/content//SMA11-4629/02-ExecutiveSummary.pdf

Substance Abuse and Mental Health Services Administration. (2012). *Screening, brief intervention, and referral to treatment (SBIRT)*. Rockville, MD: Author. Retrieved from http://www.samhsa.gov/prevention/SBIRT/index.aspx

Substance Abuse and Mental Health Services Administration–ADS Center. (2013). *SAMHSA's resource center to promote acceptance, dignity and social inclusion associated with mental health (ADS Center)*. Rockville, MD: Author. Retrieved from www.promoteacceptance.samhsa.gov/main/default.aspx

Unutzer, J., Harbin, H., Schoenbeum, M., & Druss, B. (2013). *The collaborative care model: An approach for integrating physical and mental health care in Medicaid health homes*. Retrieved from http://medicaid.gov/State-Resource-Center/Medicaid-State-Technical-Assistance/Health-Homes-Technical-Assistance/Downloads/HH-IRC-Collaborative-5-13.pdf

U.S. Surgeon General. (2001). Mental health: Culture, race and ethnicity. *Supplement to Mental health: A report to the Surgeon General*. Washington, DC: Author.

VA Healthcare Network Upstate New York. (2005). *Integrated Primary Care Behavioral Health Services Operations Manual*: VISN #2.

Van Egeren, L., & Huber, T. (n.d.). *Integrating mental health services into primary care*. Association of VA Psychologist Leaders. Retrieved from www.avapl.org/pub/PrimaryCare/MH%20PC%20Van%20Egeren.ppt

Woltmann, E., Grogan-Kaylor, A., Perron, B., Georges, H., Kilbourne, A. M., & Bauer, M. S. (2012). Comparative effectiveness of collaborative chronic care models for mental health conditions across primary, specialty, and behavioral health care settings: Systematic review and meta-analysis. *American Journal of Psychiatry, 169*, 790–804.

World Health Organization. (2007). *Integrating mental health services into primary health care*. Geneva, Switzerland: Department of Mental Health and Substance Abuse.

# The Affordable Care Act: Overview and Implications for County and City Behavioral Health and Intellectual/Developmental Disability Programs

RON MANDERSCHEID

*National Association of County Behavioral Health and Developmental Disability Directors, Washington, District of Columbia, USA*

*The author begins by reviewing the 5 key intended actions of the Affordable Care Act (ACA)—insurance reform, coverage reform, quality reform, performance reform, and information technology reform. This framework provides a basis for examining how populations served and service programs will change at the county and city levels as a result of the ACA, and how provider staff also will change over time as a result of these developments. The author concludes by outlining immediate next steps for county and city programs.*

The Affordable Care Act (ACA) holds considerable promise for improving the future of behavioral health care. Put into a historical perspective, the ACA also represents a once-in-a-century opportunity to transform our broader insurance and care systems. For these reasons, it is imperative to review the key features of the ACA and to explore their implications for the evolution of county and city behavioral health and intellectual disability and developmental disability programs. Now that President Obama has been reelected, we can expect ACA implementation to begin and proceed quickly.

As will become obvious in the discussion here, the current environment is not conducive to traditional steady-state incremental planning. Rather, we are in a period of very rapid change that demands strategic planning and design. Therefore, attention to the changes discussed here will be very important to undertake this type of planning successfully.

As a final element of context, we must note that the ACA specifically addresses social justice concerns regarding health status and care (see Braveman et al., 2011). One's health status is correlated closely with one's social class and race; hence, we find major negative health disparities, including behavioral health disparities, among persons of lower status and minority groups. These health disparities are associated with disparities in access to care. Social justice demands that we value all people equally. Thus, we need to address these class- and race-related health disparities by promoting equity in health status and care. A major focus of the ACA is the promotion of equity in health insurance coverage and care access to reduce these health disparities.

## COMPONENTS OF THE ACA

The ACA legislation is approximately 2,300 pages in length (the full act can be accessed at http://www.healthcare.gov/law/full). Almost 2,000 of those pages are devoted to insurance reform and coverage reform, the two features of the ACA that commit federal dollars. The remaining 300 pages are devoted to quality reform, performance reform, and information technology (IT) reform, all of which have been assigned to the U.S. Secretary of Health and Human Services (HHS) to implement.

A review of the major features of each of the five ACA reforms follows.

## Insurance Reform

The purpose of insurance reform is to expand health insurance coverage to approximately 32 million adult Americans who currently lack it. This will be accomplished through a Medicaid expansion, intended to cover all persons at up to 138% of the federal poverty level who currently lack health insurance, and through state health insurance exchanges, intended to cover all persons without insurance who are above 138% of the federal poverty level (estimates of the uninsured population for 2011 are available from http://www.census.gov/prod/2012pubs/p60-243.pdf).

### MEDICAID EXPANSION

This is intended to begin on January 1, 2014, and to cover about 16 million persons. Prior research indicates that about 40% of these persons—about 6.4 million—will already have a behavioral health condition at the time that they enroll, and that a majority of this latter population will have a primary

# THE AFFORDABLE CARE ACT AND INTEGRATED BEHAVIORAL HEALTH CARE

substance use condition (see an analysis at http://www.acmha.org/content/events/national/WHC_Universal_Coverage.pdf and http://www.ncbi.nlm.nih.gov/pubmed/21969638; Strine, Zack, Dhingra, Druss, & Simoes, 2011). Fully 100% of the cost of the Medicaid expansion will be paid by the federal government in 2014 through 2016, after which the federal contribution will decline to and remain at 90% by 2020.

Originally intended to be mandatory, the Medicaid expansion is now a state option as a result of the Supreme Court decision sustaining the ACA (the full text of the Supreme Court decision is available at http://www.supremecourt.gov/opinions/11pdf/11-393c3a2.pdf). However, the financial benefit to states is so considerable that most are expected to take advantage of this opportunity as soon as it becomes available. For example, because about 30% of the Texas population is currently uninsured, Texas can expect to receive about $52.5 billion in federal funds by 2020 as a result of the Medicaid expansion for a state investment of about $2.5 billion (estimates for all states are available at http://www.kff.org/healthreform/upload/medicaid-coverage-and-spending-in-health-reform-national-and-state-by-state-results-for-adults-at-or-below-133-fpl.pdf).

## STATE HEALTH INSURANCE EXCHANGES

These also are slated to begin operation on January 1, 2014. Those insured through this mechanism who are at between 139% and 400% of the federal poverty level will receive a sliding scale federal tax subsidy. Exchanges will be expected to offer a range of health insurance products, classified from bronze to platinum, and to include at least two interstate health insurance plans. The exchanges are expected to cover about 16 million persons, about a quarter of whom—about 4 million persons—will have a behavioral health condition at the time that they enroll.

About a quarter of the states currently are developing exchanges. The remaining states have various levels of indifference or opposition to the Exchange concept. After January 1, 2013, the HHS will make a determination regarding each state's readiness to implement an exchange. If the HHS determines that a state will not implement an exchange, then it will develop an exchange for that state. (The status of state exchange development as of August 2012 is available at http://statehealthfacts.kff.org/comparemaptable.jsp?ind=962&cat=17.)

The floor benefit for both the Medicaid expansion and the state health insurance exchange is the essential health benefit (EHB). This must cover 10 specific types of benefits, including mental health and substance use care and prevention. Both the mental health and the substance use benefits must be at parity with those for primary care. (A model mental health and substance use benefit is given at http://www.coalitionforwholehealth.org/2012/01/ehb-consensus-principles-and-service-recommendations/). Each state is currently defining its EHB from a benchmark health insurance plan it has chosen from among 10 options defined for it by HHS. The EHB is exceptionally important because it will define the amount of federal funds a state will receive for its Medicaid expansion and the size of the tax subsidy available to those insured under the state health insurance exchange.

## Coverage Reform

Many of the features of coverage reform have been in effect since September 23, 2010, 6 months after the signing of the ACA legislation. These features have been very well received by most Americans, because they address major deficits in our previous health insurance coverage. Here, I provide a brief overview of these changes.

### ELIMINATION OF PREEXISTING CONDITION EXCLUSIONS

Perhaps most important, no one under the age of 19 can any longer be excluded from health insurance coverage because he or she has a preexisting condition. This change was extended to all age groups on January 1, 2014.

### FAMILY COVERAGE TO AGE 26

Similarly, no one under the age of 26 can any longer be excluded from his or her family's health insurance policy.

Both of these changes have major implications for behavioral health care, as most behavioral conditions originate in the teenage years, and most behavioral health treatment first occurs in the early 20s.

### ELIMINATION OF COPAYS, DEDUCTIBLES, AND LIMITS

Disease prevention and health promotion interventions can no longer have a copay or deductible, and annual and lifetime limits for health insurance are eliminated. The latter changes have significant implications for persons suffering from major behavioral health conditions, such as schizophrenia, where family financial ruin as a result of insurance limits has been commonplace.

### INSURANCE PLAN DIRECT CARE EXPENDITURES

Other changes apply directly to insurance plans. Large insurance plans must now spend at least 85% of their revenue on care delivery, and small plans must spend at least 80% on care. Beginning in 2012, these changes have led to rebates of some insurance premiums when required thresholds were not met.

## Quality Reform

Key values around ACA quality reform include person-centered care, whole health care, and shared decision making. In other words, health care should consider all of a person's health care needs, and the person should be engaged in improving his or her health and in reducing illness (see Manderscheid, Alexandre, Everett, Leaf, & Zablotsky, 2012). Clearly, our core behavioral health concepts of whole health, wellness, resiliency, and recovery fit very well with these ACA values.

The principal tool envisioned by the ACA to improve the quality of health care is the health home. The mechanism to foster the development of a health home is an accountable care organization (ACO). Both are explained further next.

### HEALTH HOMES

Health homes integrate behavioral health care and primary care so that all of a person's health needs can be addressed through a single entity. They also offer disease prevention and health promotion interventions. Typically, they are responsible for the health care of a defined population. (One can read more about health homes at http://www.medicaid.gov/Medicaid-CHIP-Program-Information/By-Topics/Long-Term-Services-and-Support/Integrating-Care/Health-Homes/Health-Homes.html.)

Health homes relate closely to the care integration initiatives that have been pursued by the federal government and private foundations for the past half-decade. The primary motivation for these initiatives has been to provide primary care to persons with behavioral health conditions who also suffer from chronic physical illnesses, and to provide behavioral health care to persons who also have health problems. An example of the former would be diabetes care for a person who has schizophrenia; an example of the latter would be depression care for a person suffering from heart disease. Physical health conditions in public mental health clients have been found to lead to premature death and a life span shortened by as much as 25 years (Colton & Manderscheid, 2006).

### ACOs

ACOs represent the organizational arrangements being put in place to operate health homes. An ACO can be a lead organization that coordinates the activities of several subsidiary organizations, or it can be an entire new entity created specifically to operate a health home. In either case, it represents a new organizational arrangement for delivering coordinated health care and behavioral health care. (One can read more about ACOs at http://www.medicaid.gov/Federal-Policy-Guidance/downloads/SMD-12-001.pdf.)

Generally, we expect that ACOs are unlikely to be led by community behavioral health care entities, but rather by hospitals, primary care practices, federally qualified health centers, and rural health centers. Clearly, considerable field work will be necessary to integrate behavioral health care entities into ACOs.

The word *accountable* is quite significant in this context. The ACA envisions a situation in which the ACO is accountable for the health of the population it serves. Hence, the ACO will be expected to report performance measures, to be paid on an annual case or capitation basis, and to be "at risk" financially for the care delivered through the health home.

HHS has already issued field letters to announce a new state plan amendment for Medicaid programs to create health homes. Care of persons with mental illness or substance use problems is an approved focus for a state plan amendment (see this guidance at http://downloads.cms.gov/cmsgov/archived-downloads/SMDL/downloads/SMD10024.pdf). Similarly, the HHS Health Resources and Services Administration is moving quickly toward health homes through its grant programs for federally qualified health centers (FQHCs; read more about FQHCs at http://bphc.hrsa.gov/about/index.html).

## Performance Reform

Stated in simple terms, the goal of performance reform is to have all provider entities, including the new ACOs, report a small number of comparable performance measures on a periodic basis. It also is expected that these performance measures will not only reflect quality, but will also include summaries of outcomes achieved by the persons served (for a current review of outcome measures in behavioral health care and social services, see Magnabosco & Manderscheid, 2011).

These performance measures will be accompanied by changes in the manner in which care is financed. Currently, care typically is financed on a piecemeal basis, encounter by encounter. To adapt our financing mechanisms toward person-centered and whole health care, the Center for Medicare and Medicaid Services is moving Medicaid and Medicare financing systems toward annual case rates (per person served) or annual capitation rates (per person covered). A little reflection will help one realize that these are not only financing systems, but also systems to manage care that have the potential to replace traditional approaches to managed care.

## IT Reform

The ACA assumes that provider entities, such as ACOs, already have and are using electronic health records (EHRs) in a meaningful way. Thus, the ACA encourages their use through financial incentives. For example, if an entity reports its performance measures to the federal government using EHRs, it will receive a federal financial incentive.

Because behavioral health care entities were virtually excluded from American Recovery and Reinvestment Act funds allocated to provider entities to develop EHRs, an effort currently is underway to extend these grant funds to behavioral health care. Senate Resolution S-539 and House Resolution HR-6043 were introduced in 2012 to remedy this problem. Further action on these resolutions is expected before the end of the 2012 Congress (read S-538 at http://thomas.loc.gov/cgi-bin/query/z?c112:S.539; read HR-6043 at http://thomas.loc.gov/cgi-bin/query/z?c112:H.R.6043).

## POPULATION AND SERVICE IMPLICATIONS FOR COUNTY AND CITY PROGRAMS

Both the Medicaid expansion and the state health insurance exchanges will have a considerable effect on the populations served by county and city behavioral health care and intellectual and developmental disability programs.

- First, we expect that the numbers of adults served will grow considerably, beginning on January 1, 2014.
- Second, we expect that the relative balance of this new adult service population will favor persons with primary substance use conditions.
- Third, we expect that uninsured children will be identified through the adult health insurance enrollment process, that they will become newly insured either through Medicaid or through the state children's health insurance program, and that a subset will enter the public behavioral health service population.
- Fourth, we expect that a set of previously uninsured adults with intellectual and developmental disabilities will be identified and become insured.

Clear implications exist for county and city programs.

- First, it will be exceptionally important to develop an understanding in advance about the characteristics of the anticipated new service population: What are the demographic characteristics? The clinical characteristics? The service needs?
- Second, at the appropriate time, it also will be very important to help these people enroll in the new insurance programs. Software tools will be made available by HHS for this purpose.
- Third, many of these new service users will need to be taught how a behavioral health care clinic operates and how to access care through a clinic.

County and city service programs also will need to change. Likely, there will be at least two phases to this transformation:

1. First, programs will need to adapt not only to the behavioral health and intellectual and developmental disability needs of newly insured persons, but also to their social service needs. We can expect that many newly insured persons in the Medicaid expansion will come from among the homeless population and the jail population. At the same time, service programs will need to adapt so that they can offer disease prevention and health promotion interventions to those with behavioral health service needs, as well as to newly insured persons who do not have behavioral health conditions.
2. Second, county and city program directors will need to begin planning for the introduction of health homes and ACOs. Initially, this might involve improvements to coordinated care for public services. Subsequently, counties and cities might wish to take the lead in forming and providing oversight for ACOs that operate health homes. Although this latter topic is very important going forward, further development here is beyond the scope of this article.

## STAFFING IMPLICATIONS FOR COUNTY AND CITY PROGRAMS

At present, it is crucial for county and city programs to identify a strategy officer or strategy workgroup who will assume responsibility for helping to adapt these programs into the new demands of the ACA. Such a person or group should be able to collaborate easily outside the organization and be sensitive to changes occurring in that environment. Of great importance, this person or group also must be able to translate these external changes into organizational strategies and actions that help the organization work more effectively with external partners. The ACA era is expected to be characterized by collaboration and partnerships, rather than by solitary action.

Because of the anticipated expansion of the service population, even in the short term, county and city organizations will need to expand their workforce rapidly to accommodate the newly emerging demands. Peer supporters represent a readily available workforce that is well suited to undertake the new tasks that will be required. Peer supporters will be able to help the new clients navigate the Medicaid expansion and the state health insurance exchange, and to enroll in health insurance. They also will be able to help these new clients navigate access to care and will provide necessary support based on their personal experiences (Davidson, Chinman, Sells, & Rowe, 2006).

Another potential resource pool is comprised of primary care providers in the community. These could be providers from the local hospital, health center, or primary care practice. Many of these providers have developed expertise serving behavioral health clients, and they might be willing to make these skills available to county or city programs. Currently, about 60% of behavioral health care services are provided by primary care practitioners (see further details in Wang et al., 2005).

Finally, greater reliance will need to be placed on IT tools used to conduct assessments and deliver care. Such tools can range from phone apps, to in-office assessments, to telemedicine at a distance, to online cognitive-behavioral therapy. Feasibility work should be undertaken right now to determine which are most suitable.

## IMMEDIATE NEXT STEPS

The very best way to characterize the immediate next steps is for county and city programs to answer the following four questions:

1. Have we undertaken intensive strategic planning for implementing the ACA?
2. Have we identified and initiated discussions with potential partner organizations in the community?
3. Have we developed an understanding of the personal and clinical characteristics of the newly insured service population?
4. Have we begun to identify and address our future staffing needs?

The ACA provides a wonderful opportunity to address many intractable behavioral health care problems in our communities. We will only be able to take advantage of this opportunity if we prepare effectively right now.

Good luck on this exciting journey!

## REFERENCES

Braveman, P. A., Kumanyika, S., Fielding, J., LaVeist, T., Borrell, L. N., Manderscheid, R., & Troutman, A. (2011). Health disparities and health equity: The issue is justice. *American Journal of Public Health*, *101*(S1), S149–S155. doi:10.2105/AJPH.2010.3000062.

Colton, C. W., & Manderscheid, R. W. (2006). Congruencies in increased mortality rates, years of potential life lost, and causes of death in public mental health clients in eight states. *Prevention of Chronic Disease*, *3*(2), A42. Retrieved from http://www.cdc.gov/pcd/issues/2006/apr/05_0160.htm

Davidson, L., Chinman, M., Sells, D., & Rowe, M. (2006). Peer support among adults with serious mental illness: A report from the field. *Schizophrenia Bulletin*, *32*, 443–450.

Magnabosco, J. L., & Manderscheid, R. W. (Eds.). (2011). *Outcome measurement in the human services: Cross-cutting issues and methods in the era of health reform*. Washington, DC: NASW Press.

Manderscheid, R. W., Alexandre, P., Everett, A., Leaf, P., & Zablotsky, B. (2012). American mental health services: Perspective through care patterns for 100 adults, with aggregate facility, service, and cost estimates. In W. E. Eaton (Ed.), *Public mental health* (pp. 381–395). Oxford, UK: Oxford University Press.

Strine, T. W., Zack, M., Dhingra, S., Druss, B., & Simoes, E. (2011). Uninsurance among nonelderly adults with and without frequent mental and physical distress in the United States. *Psychiatric Services, 62,* 1131–1137.

Wang, P. S., Lane, M., Olfson, M., Pincus, H. A., Wells, K. B., & Kessler, R. C. (2005). Twelve-month use of mental health services in the United States: Results from the National Comorbidity Survey Replication. *Archives of General Psychiatry, 62,* 629–640.

# State *Olmstead* Litigation and the Affordable Care Act

TERENCE NG, ALICE WONG, and CHARLENE HARRINGTON

*Department of Social & Behavioral Sciences, University of California, San Francisco, San Francisco, California, USA*

*Over the past two decades, major efforts have been undertaken to expand access to Medicaid home and community-based services (HCBS) for the elderly and disabled. Despite this, many states still have long waiting lists for HCBS. Using data collected, this study examined the trends in* Olmstead *and related cases against states between 1999 and 2011. The findings show there were 131 cases filed during the period, and 90 cases were resolved through court rulings and settlements. These court cases have played an important role in encouraging states to expand access to HCBS programs and to transfer individuals out of institutions.*

In 1995, litigation was brought against the Georgia State Commissioner of Human Resources (Tommy Olmstead) on behalf of two women with developmental disabilities and mental illness (known as L.C. and E.W.; Atlanta Legal Aid Society, 2004). After voluntary admission to the Georgia Regional Hospital psychiatric unit, they eventually indicated a preference for discharge and professionals assessed that they were able to move into a community setting with appropriate support. After the patients' unsuccessful efforts to be discharged, the Atlanta Legal Aid Society brought the lawsuit on their behalf, eventually heard by the Supreme Court. The U.S. Supreme Court's decision in *Olmstead v. L.C.* (1999) was that the women had the right to receive care in the most integrated setting appropriate and that their unnecessary institutionalization was discriminatory and violated Title II of the Americans with Disabilities Act (ADA, 1990; *Olmstead v. L.C.*, 1999).

The *Olmstead* ruling held that public entities are required to provide community-based services under three conditions: (a) when the services are appropriate, (b) the affected persons do not oppose community-based treatment, and (c) when the community services can be reasonably accommodated (*Olmstead v. L.C.*, 1999). The *Olmstead* Supreme Court ruling ushered in a series of new litigation cases that have had an impact on state Medicaid programs, along with related legal cases filed under the Rehabilitation Act (1973), which also requires living in the most integrated setting, and the Medicaid law (U.S. Department of Justice, 2006, 2011a, 2011b; U.S. Department of Justice, Office of Civil Rights, 2005). Many lawsuits have focused on whether the state is making enough effort (e.g., financial and administrative commitment) and whether states are providing adequate access to home and community-based services (HCBS) with "reasonable promptness," as required by the Social Security Act §1902(a)(8) (1965). Legal arguments often focus on whether states have developed a comprehensive *Olmstead* plan with "measurable goals" and "specific timeframes" for moving people out of institutions, and evidence of active engagement and progress toward more community-integrated long-term care (Rosenbaum & Teitelbaum, 2004; Smith & Calandrillo, 2001).

This article describes the various programs that states use to provide Medicaid HCBS and some of the state and federal initiatives to expand access. Unfortunately the demand for services has been growing and many states have waiting lists for individuals who need HCBS services. This article presents data collected from web-based searches to examine the trends in *Olmstead* and related cases against states between 1999 and 2011. These court cases have played an important role in encouraging states to expand access to HCBS programs and to transfer individuals out of institutions. The discussion describes some new initiatives under the Affordable Care Act that might help states expand their HCBS programs to better address the growing demand for services and to avoid further *Olmstead* litigations.


## MEDICAID HOME- AND COMMUNITY-BASED SERVICES

There are three main programs that states use to provide Medicaid HCBS: (a) the mandatory home health benefit, (b) the optional state plan personal care services benefit, and (c) optional 1915(c) HCBS waivers. In addition, some states have implemented HCBS programs under 1115 waivers for research and demonstration projects.

Medicaid home health is a mandatory state plan benefit for individuals aged 21 and older who are entitled to, but not necessarily eligible for, nursing home care with mainly posthospital skilled nursing services. Home health is offered by all states and serves all Medicaid adult population groups (Ng, Harrington, & Kitchener, 2010). In 2009, 975,929 persons were served in all 51 home health programs across the nation at a cost of more than $5.3 billion (Ng & Harrington, 2012).

The personal care services (PCS) program was established in 1975 (under Section 1905(24) of the Social Security Act) to allow for a Medicaid state plan optional benefit to provide assistance with activities of daily living (ADLs; e.g., bathing and dressing) and instrumental activities of daily living (IADLs; e.g., preparing meals and shopping; Ng et al., 2010; U.S. Department of Health & Human Services, 2010). In 2009, 912,076 persons were served in 32 state plan personal care programs at a cost of almost $11 billion (Ng & Harrington, 2012).

Since 1981, states have used the authority under Section 1915(c) of the Social Security Act to waive certain federal Medicaid requirements (including comparability in amount, duration, or scope of services and in state-wideness) to establish HCBS waiver programs (Ng et al., 2010; U.S. Department of Health and Human Services, 2010). These programs attract federal matching funds and allow states to provide a wide range of HCBS to participants who would otherwise qualify for an institutional level of care. In 2009, the 1915(c) waiver program was the largest HCBS Medicaid program, with 1,329,235 persons served in 286 waivers across 48 states and Washington, DC, at a cost of more than $33 billion (Ng & Harrington, 2012).

In programs where demand exceeds the allocated slots, states are allowed to establish waiting lists, which can slow deinstitutionalization of individuals out of nursing homes and into the home and community and can limit access to services for those in the community. In spite of the expansion of HCBS programs across the states, there is a growing demand for HCBS that states have not been able to meet. In 2011, there were 511,174 persons on waiver waiting lists, where the average waiting time is 25 months for waiver services (Ng & Harrington, 2012). States have reported that their waiting lists have increased from 192,447 in 2002 to more than 511,000 in 2011. In addition, states may also place added limitations on HCBS provisions and waiver services as a way of controlling costs. When such limitations on services increase the risk of a person's institutionalization, plaintiffs are entitled to seek the court's help under *Olmstead*'s "reasonable effort" theory.


## INITIATIVES TO EXPAND HCBS PROGRAMS

To help states comply with the *Olmstead* ruling, the Centers for Medicare and Medicaid Services (CMS, 2010) have initiated many actions since 2000. These include issuing state guidance based on legal opinions and encouraging review and development of state *Olmstead* plans and programs that expand Medicaid 1915(c) HCBS waivers and PCS, along with greater flexibility in

Medicaid HCBS waiver programs (Carlson & Coffey, 2010; Fox-Grage, Folkemer, & Lewis, 2004). By 2011, just over half the states (26) had developed *Olmstead* plans, 18 states reported alternative responses, and 7 states had neither (Ng, Wong, & Harrington, 2011a, 2011b; Rosenbaum & Teitelbaum, 2004).

CMS awarded Real Choice Systems Change Grants for Community Living to improve state infrastructures from 2000 through 2009. Nursing facility transition grants were started in 2001 and the Money Follows the Person demonstrations were established in 2003 and extended under the Deficit Reduction Act (DRA) of 2005 and the Patient Protection and Affordable Care Act (ACA, 2010; Carlson & Coffey, 2010; Kassner et al., 2008; Ng, Harrington, & Musumeci, 2011). The DRA also allowed states to move waiver programs into a new HCBS state plan benefit (Section 1915(i) of the Social Security Act) and expanded the Cash and Counseling program (1915(j) state plan option; Carlson & Coffey, 2010; Kassner et al., 2008; Ng, Harrington, & Musumeci, 2011). Other federal programs were initiated to improve HCBS, transform mental health systems, integrate long-term supports with affordable housing, and reduce the reliance on institutional care (Kassner et al., 2008).

The many federal and state initiatives have resulted in a steady increase in Medicaid HCBS participants and expenditures. In 2009, there were a total of 3.2 million participants in Medicaid HCBS programs, having increased from fewer than 1 million since 1999 (Ng & Harrington, 2012). Overall spending on Medicaid HCBS increased from $17 billion in 1999 to over $49 billion in 2009, although wide variation in participants and expenditures occurred across states (Ng & Harrington, 2012).

States can also deliver HCBS through the Medicaid state plan or through Section 1115 Research and Demonstration waivers (Artiga, 2011). These waivers have been used as a vehicle to implement programs such as cash and counseling, personal care payment for spouses, independence plus, and managed care waivers. In 2011, 30 states and the District of Columbia had approved Section 1115 waivers for managed care, 12 states had existing Medicaid managed care long-term services and supports (MLTSS) programs, and another 11 states have plans for implementation in the next 2 years (Cheek et al., 2012). Another report noted that MLTSS grew from 8 states in 2004 to 16 states in 2012, and the numbers of persons served increased from 105,000 to 389,000 (Saucier, Kasten, Burwell, & Gold, 2012).

## STUDY DATA AND METHODS

### Data Sources

This study on *Olmstead* litigation used two research strategies: (a) a primary Web-based search on lawsuits, and (b) a search of secondary studies from legal, health care, and disability sources. For the primary search, we collected data from legal databases (e.g., LexisNexis) and organizations involved in the lawsuits. The primary research was used to identify new litigation cases and resolutions and to clarify information about previously identified lawsuits. The secondary searches covered five domains: journals, databases, authors, keywords, and organizations. Using multiple secondary sources avoided duplication of previous work and collated existing information in an accessible way, but this approach depends on the accuracy of secondary sources. Where details about lawsuits were inconsistent, we used legal databases as the primary source.

Although we excluded lawsuits that were decided before the *Olmstead* ruling in 1999 from detailed analysis, relevant pre-1999 community integration-type cases were used for pre- and post-*Olmstead* comparisons. Cases that were initiated before the *Olmstead* case was decided but were resolved after 1999 were included. We included related *Olmstead* litigation if it was resolved in 1999 or later.

## Data Analysis

Legal cases were classified as (a) *Olmstead* cases, and (b) *Olmstead*-related cases. *Olmstead* cases were those about people who are institutionalized or at risk of institutionalization that cited a violation of the ADA Title II. *Olmstead*-related cases were those that did not cite the ADA but used another law such as the Medicaid law or the Rehabilitation Act. We classified cases into those that were closed and those that were active or continuing cases during 2011. In addition, we classified cases by their client target groups: physically disabled, mentally retarded or developmentally disabled, mentally ill, and combination diagnosis or others that included persons with traumatic brain injury or with AIDS. We identified the specific litigation activities undertaken by the U.S. Department of Justice, individual plaintiffs, or class action cases. We also categorized the number of cases by state and by year, and summarized all the cases that were completed prior to 1999. Finally, we examined the outcome of each case in terms of court rulings, settlements, or continuations.

## STUDY FINDINGS

Between 1999 and December 2011, there were a total of 131 *Olmstead* and related lawsuits filed in courts. This averaged about 10 cases a year in the 13 years after the *Olmstead* decision. In contrast, there were a total of 51 cases in the years before 1999, after the first case was filed in 1970. Figure 1 shows that there was a spike in cases filed immediately after the *Olmstead* ruling, but this leveled off and there were no cases filed in 2007. The number of cases grew again in 2009 and 2010.

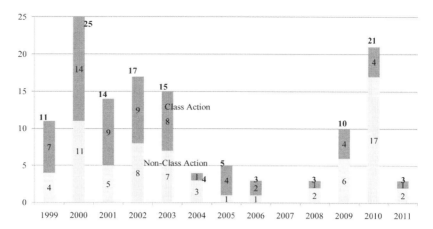

**FIGURE 1** Number of class action and non-class-action *Olmstead* and related cases filed in the United States, 1999–2011.

A case might be granted class action status by the presiding judge if the number of persons seeking relief is too numerous to hear individually, if the harm suffered is similar, and if the relief sought is similar (U.S. Department of Justice, Office of Civil Rights, 2005). Defendants usually do not want to face a class action suit because they would have to provide relief and compensation to a large number of people if they lose. On the other hand, plaintiffs might prefer a class action certification to reduce the cost and number of lawsuits against the same party and to allow them to seek better terms in settlement negotiations.

Between 1999 and 2011, almost half (64 cases) of the 131 total lawsuits were granted class action status (Figure 1). This shows that many of these cases involved a large number of persons who might have been denied HCBS or lacked sufficient HCBS to prevent institutionalization. A majority of the *Olmstead* and related class action cases were settled before a verdict was handed down. Almost 47% of all cases filed before *Olmstead* (in 1999) were also class action cases. The *Olmstead* ruling did not spur an increase in class action cases, but did increase the overall number of cases. Among the 64 total class action lawsuits filed in this period, 47 of them were closed with either a settlement or a verdict. It takes an average of 2.8 years for such cases to close, with a case in California lasting 7 years. The 67 non-class-action cases took an average of 2.1 years to come to a conclusion, with the longest case being in Washington, lasting 9 years.

Out of a total 131 *Olmstead* and related cases filed since 1999, most states had at least one *Olmstead* or related case. Three states (California, Illinois, and Pennsylvania) had 10 cases each, Florida and Washington had 8, and Arkansas and New York had 5 cases each. Eight states did not have any post-*Olmstead* cases (Idaho, Iowa, North Dakota, South Dakota, Wyoming, Vermont, Rhode Island, and Maryland). Only Iowa, North Dakota,

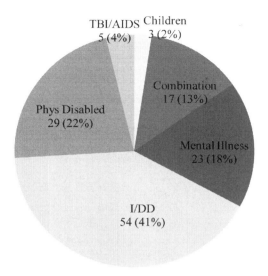

**FIGURE 2** *Olmstead* and related cases by target group, 1999–2011. TBI/AIDS = traumatic brain injury/Acquired Immune Deficiency Syndrome; I/DD = intellectually or developmentally disabled.

South Dakota, and Vermont were never involved in an *Olmstead* or related case before or after 1999.

Figure 2 shows that among the 131 *Olmstead* and related cases filed between 1999 and 2011, almost 60% were filed by plaintiffs who were diagnosed as intellectually or developmentally disabled or with mental illness. More than 10% of cases were filed by persons with different diagnoses and needs that we labeled as a combination target group. The fact that individuals with intellectual or developmental disabilities made up 41% of individuals in Medicaid HCBS waiver programs but 63% of individuals on HCBS waiting lists might explain the high percentage of legal actions taken by this group (Howard, Ng, & Harrington, 2011).

No specific elderly target group was reported, although elderly individuals might be included within the physically disabled or the combination group. Because elderly and disabled individuals represented 48% of Medicaid 1915c waiver participants, the lack of legal cases could imply that elderly persons are less likely to seek legal help or that there are sufficient HCBS provisions for them (Howard et al., 2011).

Before 1999, almost two-thirds of all cases were filed by persons with either intellectual or developmental disabilities or mental illness and 16% were filed by persons with physical disability. Therefore, the types of individuals filing cases were about the same in the post-*Olmstead* period.

Before *Olmstead*, 42 out of a total of 51 resolved cases (82%) were either settled or won by the plaintiff. Only 9 cases were won by defendants (see Table 1). After *Olmstead*, there was a similar trend, with 76 out of 90 resolved

## THE AFFORDABLE CARE ACT AND INTEGRATED BEHAVIORAL HEALTH CARE

**TABLE 1** Outcomes of *Olmstead* and Related Cases, Pre-1999 to 2011

|  | Pre-1999 | 1999 | 2000 | 2001 | 2002 | 2003 | 2004 | 2005 | 2006 | 2007 | 2008 | 2009 | 2010 | 2011 | Total |
|---|---|---|---|---|---|---|---|---|---|---|---|---|---|---|---|
| Settlement | 25 | 5 | 16 | 7 | 10 | 7 | 2 | 3 | 2 | 0 | 0 | 4 | 4 | 1 | 86 |
| Plaintiff win | 17 | 3 | 4 | 2 | 1 | 1 | 0 | 0 | 0 | 0 | 1 | 1 | 2 | 0 | 32 |
| Defendant win | 9 | 2 | 3 | 1 | 2 | 2 | 0 | 0 | 0 | 0 | 0 | 2 | 2 | 0 | 23 |

cases (84%) either settled or won by the plaintiff. A settlement agreement was the most likely outcome for cases with 86 out of a total of 141 resolved cases being settled (61%) over the pre- and post-*Olmstead* period. A settlement is an out-of-court negotiation and agreement that avoids a court verdict, which avoids costly, drawn-out court hearings and usually takes into account the needs of both parties.

Some of the class action cases have affected large numbers of individuals. For example, in *Ligas et al. v Hamos et al.* (Center for Personal Assistance Services Illinois Olmstead Cases, 2013) in Illinois, nine plaintiffs obtained class certification for persons living in private state-funded intermediate care facilities for the developmentally disabled (ICF-DD's) or who were at risk of entering such facilities when they sought HCBS but were denied by the state (Equip for Equality, 2011). The state settled the case in 2011 by agreeing to provide timely evaluations and transitions to integrated community settings for about 6,000 persons living in ICF-MR facilities. In addition, over a 6-year period, 3,000 people with developmental disabilities who were living at home without services were to be given community services. An independent monitor with expertise in developmental disabilities was appointed by the court to oversee the implementation and compliance with the settlement agreement.

Another class action *Olmstead* lawsuit was *Capitol People First et al. v. CA Dept of Developmental Services et al.*, (Center for Personal Assistance Services California Olmstead Cases, 2013a) which was granted final settlement approval in 2009. Sixteen plaintiffs filed a lawsuit to compel California to provide HCBS information and options to institutionalized persons in 2002. After class certification was obtained for more than 7,000 persons living in large state institutions (e.g., state hospitals and skilled nursing facilities), a settlement agreement was reached in 2009. The settlement obligated the state to provide relevant and timely information about transitions to smaller, community-based settings for persons in large institutions and new community programs and housing to accommodate the transition into HCBS settings for class members (Disability Rights California, 2011).

A smaller Olmstead lawsuit was *Chambers et al. v. City of San Francisco* (Center for Personal Assistance Services California Olmstead Cases, 2013b) which was granted final settlement approval in 2008. The lead plaintiff in the case, Chambers, had been a resident of Laguna Honda Hospital in San Francisco since 1999 and wanted to live in the community. This settlement benefited at least 500 persons by establishing an assessment and coordination of care system with access to a Medi-Cal HCBS waiver, a rental subsidy program for affordable and accessible housing, and attendant and nursing care, mental health services, assistance with meals, and substance abuse treatment (Gershon, 2008).

## DISCUSSION

These *Olmstead* cases show the importance of litigation for many persons with disabilities who want to obtain Medicaid HCBS and avoid unnecessary institutionalization, ruled as discriminatory more than a decade ago. Institutional bias in Medicaid long-term care occurs because nursing home and institutional services are mandatory, whereas HCBS programs are optional and states are allowed to limit the services available. This contributes to inadequate access to and availability of HCBS for persons with disabilities.

Although the litigation process has largely been successful, most of the cases take a few years (an average of 3 years) to complete and if the plaintiffs win a court verdict or a settlement agreement, the implementation often takes a few years. For vulnerable individuals who are forced into institutional care during this process, the delayed litigation process might not directly benefit many of those who filed the cases. Moreover, the cost of such litigation and the length of time required before the resolution of such cases means that many institutionalized persons with disabilities are deterred from redress through the courts.

One study contends that "*Olmstead*'s legacy in the courts has been uneven" due to the subjectivity involved in deciding whether changes sought by plaintiffs to a state Medicaid program constitute a fundamental alteration (Rosenbaum & Teitelbaum, 2004; Rosenbaum, Teitelbaum, & Stewart, 2001). On the other hand, the use of litigation to increase deinstitutionalization and community integration of people has clearly been a catalyst to stimulate long-term care reforms (Enbar, Morris, Miller, & Naiditch, 2004).

Numerous barriers exist to implementing *Olmstead* plans and promoting the inclusion of people with disabilities in the community. Financial constraints on Medicaid and political pressures to maintain institutional facilities are the major problems states could face when implementing their *Olmstead* plans (Kaiser Family Foundation Policy Brief, 2004). Other systemic barriers are (a) regulatory and financing restrictions and inadequate infrastructure in the areas of housing, workforce, service flexibility, and information management; (b) inadequate public awareness of community-based options; and (c) lack of consumer involvement in the design, implementation, and monitoring of state *Olmstead* responses (Chaney, 2003). Although progress has been made on *Olmstead* planning, continued efforts and initiatives are necessary for states to continue to fully implement their plans (Chaney, 2003).

The ACA legislation of 2010 included a number of provisions aimed at addressing Medicaid's continuing institutional bias (Patient Protection & Affordable Care Act, 2010). States have three new or modified options that can be used to expand Medicaid HCBS programs and help rebalance their participants and expenditures: (a) the State Balancing Incentive Program, (b) the Community First Choice Option, and (c) HCBS as a State Plan benefit. The ACA also extended mandatory spousal impoverishment protections to community-based spouses of people receiving HCBS, authorized additional funds for aging disability and resource centers, and extended the Money Follows the Person Demonstration (Harrington, Ng, LaPlante, & Kaye, 2012).

The State Balancing Incentive Program helps states to increase their share of MLTSS spending on HCBS while reducing their share of MLTSS spending on institutional care through enhanced matching federal funding for HCBS. The Community First Choice Option is a new Medicaid state plan benefit that provides self-directed, community-based attendant supports and services (e.g., personal care) to certain individuals with disabilities. States that take up this option receive an enhanced federal matching rate of 6%. HCBS as a State Plan Benefit allows states to provide HCBS to individuals with incomes up to 150% of the federal poverty level who are Medicaid eligible under a group covered by the state plan, without regard to whether individuals meet an institutional level of care (Ng, Harrington, & Musumeci, 2011). This benefit will help states to cover all eligible persons in their states rather than limited categories of participants that are required through the 1915(c) waiver. It will also help states avoid HCBS wait list *Olmstead* lawsuits, as this benefit disallows wait lists for services.

Although the new initiatives can help states in expanding access to HCBS programs, states continue to face fiscal constraints that limit their ability to fund the new programs. States could also take a look-and-see attitude when applying for and implementing these initiatives, as these new programs are optional and might increase overall Medicaid long-term care expenditures if there is a "woodwork" effect that increases participation.

In conclusion, as the number of *Olmstead* cases against states mount, the growing waiting lists for HCBS mean that access to Medicaid HCBS has not kept pace with the increased demand for HCBS. However, new initiations within the ACA might help reduce institutionalization and HCBS wait lists due to provisions within the ACA that encourage states to expand HCBS and eliminate wait lists. There might still be a need for consumers to resort to *Olmstead* litigation in certain states, as it is often a critical step in forcing states to transition individuals to the home and community and to increase access to HCBS.

## FUNDING

This research was funded by the National Institute on Disability and Rehabilitation Research (Grant No. H133B080002). The views expressed in this article are those of the authors and do not necessarily reflect those of the sponsors.

## REFERENCES

Americans with Disabilities Act of 1990, 42 U.S.C. § 1210(b)(1).

Artiga, S. (2011). *Five key questions and answers about Section 1115 Medicaid Demonstration Waivers*. Washington, DC: Kaiser Commission on Medicaid and the Uninsured.

Atlanta Legal Aid Society. (2004). Olmstead v. LC *and EW landmark case*. Atlanta, GA: Author. Retrieved from http://www.atlantalegalaid.org/impact.htm

Carlson, E., & Coffey, G. (2010). *10-plus years after the* Olmstead *ruling: Progress, problems, and opportunities*. Washington, DC: National Senior Citizens Law Center.

Center for Personal Assistance Services California Olmstead Cases (2013a). Capitals People First et al. v. CA Dept. of Departmental Services et al.

Center for Personal Assistance Services California Olmstead Cases (2013b). Mark Chambers et al. v. City and Country of San Francisco.

Center for Personal Assistance Services Illinois Olmstead Cases (2013). Ligas et al. v. Hamos et al. 05-CV-4331.

Centers for Medicare & Medicaid Services. (2010, May). *Community living initiative* (State Medicaid Director Letter, SMDL No. 10-008). Baltimore, MD: Author. Retrieved from http://www.cms.gov/smdl/downloads/SMD10008.pdf

Chaney, R. (2003). *Promoting community integration: Barriers and best practices from seven state recipients of* Olmstead *planning grants*. Washington, DC: Center for Health Care Strategies.

Cheek, M., Roherty, M., Finnan, L., Cho, E., Walls, J., Gifford, K., . . . Ujvari, K. (2012). *On the verge: The transformation of long term services and supports*. Washington, DC: AARP Public Policy Institute. Retrieved from http://www.aarp.org/health/ health-care-reform/info-02-2012/On-the-Verge-The-Transformation-of-Long-Term-Services-and-Supports-AARP-ppi-ltc.html

Defecit Reduction Act of 2005, Pub. L. 109–171 (2005).

Disability Rights California. (2011). *Community living lawsuit*—Capitol People First v. DDS. Sacramento, CA: Author. Retrieved from http://www.disabilityrightsca. org/advocacy/cpfvdds/index.htm

Enbar, E. G., Morris, A. F., Miller, L., & Naiditch, Z. (2004). *A nationwide study of deinstitutionalization & community integration: A special report of the public policy and legal advocacy programs*. Chicago, IL: Equip for Equality. Retrieved from http://www.equipforequality.org/publications/cipp_final.doc

Equip for Equality. (2011). *Documents relevant to* Ligas v. Maram—*Lawsuit seeking community services for people with developmental disabilities in Illinois*. Chicago, IL: Author. Retrieved from http://equipforequality.org/news/pressreleases/ ligasmaramfiles.php

Fox-Grage, W., Folkemer, D., & Lewis, J. (2004). *The states' response to the* Olmstead *decision: How are states complying? A 2003 update.* Washington, DC: National Conference of State Legislatures.

Gershon, E. (2008). *Groundbreaking settlement in San Francisco: New housing and community services created for seniors and adults with disabilities.* Oakland, CA: Protection & Advocacy, Inc. Retrieved from http://jfactivist.typepad.com/jfactivist/2008/09/groundbreaking.html

Harrington, C., Ng, T., LaPlante, M., & Kaye, C. (2012). Medicaid home and community based service: Impact of the PPACA. *Journal of Aging & Social Policy, 24,* 169–187.

Howard, J., Ng, T., & Harrington, C. (2011). *Medicaid home and community based service programs: Data update* (Report prepared for the Kaiser Commission on Medicaid and the Uninsured). Washington, DC: Kaiser Commission on Medicaid and the Uninsured. Retrieved from http://www.kff.org/medicaid/upload/7720-05.pdf

Kaiser Family Foundation Policy Brief. (2004). Olmstead v. L.C.: *The interaction of the Americans with Disabilities Act and Medicaid.* Washington, DC: Kaiser Commission on Medicaid and the Uninsured. Retrieved from http://www.kff.org/medicaid/7096a.cfm

Kassner, E., Reinhard, S., Fox-Grage, W., Houser, A., Accius, J., Coleman, B., & Milne, D. (2008). *A balancing act: State long-term care reform.* Washington, DC: AARP Public Policy Institute. Retrieved from www.aarp.org/ppi

Ng, T., & Harrington, C. (2012). *Medicaid home and community-based service programs: 2009 data update* (Report prepared for the Kaiser Commission on Medicaid & the Uninsured). Washington, DC: Kaiser Commission on Medicaid & the Uninsured.

Ng, T., Harrington, C., & Kitchener, M. (2010). Medicare and Medicaid in long-term care. *Health Affairs, 29,* 22–28.

Ng, T., Harrington, C., & Musumeci, M. (2011). *State options that expand access to Medicaid home and community-based services.* Washington, DC: Kaiser Commission on Medicaid & the Uninsured. Retrieved from http://www.kff.org/medicaid/8241.cfm

Ng, T., Wong, A., & Harrington, C. (2011a). *Home and community based services: Introduction to* Olmstead *lawsuits and* Olmstead *plans.* San Francisco, CA: Center for Personal Assistance Services. Retrieved from http://www.pascenter.org/olmstead/

Ng, T., Wong, A., & Harrington, C. (2011b). Olmstead *and* Olmstead *related lawsuits.* San Francisco, CA: Center for Personal Assistance Services. Retrieved from http://www.pascenter.org/olmstead/olmsteadcases.php

Olmstead v. L. C., 527 U.S. 581 (1999). Retrieved from http://www.law.cornell.edu/supct/html/98-536.ZS.html

Patient Protection and Affordable Care Act, Pub. L. No. 111–148, 124 Stat. 119 (2010).

Rehabilitation Act of 1973, amended 1993 and 1998, Pub. L. No. 93–112, 87 Stat. 355.

Rosenbaum, S., & Teitelbaum, J. (2004). Olmstead *at five: Assessing the impact.* Washington, DC: Kaiser Commission on Medicaid & the Uninsured. Retrieved from http://www.kff.org/medicaid/7105a.cfm

Rosenbaum, S., Teitelbaum, J., & Stewart, A. (2001). *An analysis of* Olmstead *complaints: Implications for policy and long-term planning.* Washington, DC: Center for Health Care Strategies.

Saucier, P., Kasten, J., Burwell, B., & Gold, L. (2012). *The growth of managed long-term services and supports (MLTSS) programs: A 2012 update.* Ann Arbor, MI: Truven Health Analytics.

Social Security Act Title XIX of 1965, Section 1902 [42 U.S.C. 1396a] (a) (8) (1965).

Smith, J. D. E., & Calandrillo, S. P. (2001). Forward to fundamental alteration: Addressing ADA Title II integration lawsuits after *Olmstead v. L.C. Harvard Journal of Law & Public Policy, 24,* 695. Retrieved from http://papers.ssrn.com/sol3/papers.cfm?abstract_id=694002

U.S. Department of Health and Human Services, Office of the Assistant Secretary for Planning & Evaluation. (2010). *Understanding Medicaid home and community services: A primer* (2010 edition). Washington, DC: Assistant Secretary for Planning & Evaluation.

U.S. Department of Justice. (2006). *Delivering on the promise: OCR's compliance activities promote community integration.* Washington, DC: Author. Retrieved from http://www.hhs.gov/ocr/civilrights/resources/specialtopics/community/deliveringonthepromisereport.html

U.S. Department of Justice. (2011a). Olmstead *litigation in the 12 U.S. Circuit Courts of Appeals.* Washington, DC: Author. Retrieved from http://www.ada.gov/olmstead/olmstead_enforcement.htm

U.S. Department of Justice. (2011b). *Statement of the Department of Justice on enforcement of the integration mandate of Title II of the Americans with Disabilities Act and* Olmstead v. L.C. Washington, DC: Author. Retrieved from http://www.ada.gov/olmstead/

U.S. Department of Justice, Office of Civil Rights. (2005). *A guide to disability rights laws.* Washington, DC: Author. Retrieved from http://www.ada.gov/cguide.htm

# The Affordable Care Act for Behavioral Health Consumers and Families

### TED J. JOHNSON

*Allied Health, Kanawha Valley Community and Technical College, South Charleston, West Virginia, USA*

### DAVID H. SANDERS

*Psychiatric Rehabilitation Association, Charleston, West Virginia, USA*

### JUDY L. STANGE

*Magna Systems, Inc., Alexandria, Virginia, USA*

*The Affordable Care Act (ACA) is legislation that might ultimately make health insurance coverage available to all Americans. The ACA is scheduled for full implementation in 2014. Many decisions are still being made concerning implementation. Provisions of the ACA are of paramount importance to persons with mental illnesses and substance use disorders. This is a brief overview of key elements of the ACA and potential effects on consumers of behavioral health services and their families. Behavioral health consumers and their families include persons with mental illnesses, as well as persons with substance use disorders, and their families.*

The Patient Protection and Affordable Care Act (ACA) was signed into law March 23, 2010, by President Barack Obama and the key elements of the Act were upheld in a U.S. Supreme Court decision issued in 2012. The ACA was expected to expand health insurance coverage to about 32 million newly covered individuals, with about half of that number to be covered by

Medicaid, and the other half through private insurance that can be purchased by individuals with cost offsets through tax credits. Approximately 4 to 6 million individuals among the newly covered were expected to need treatment for mental health and substance abuse disorders. Although the original intent of the ACA was to require all states to expand Medicaid to serve this population, the Supreme Court decision granted states the option to expand or not expand their Medicaid program.

At the time of this writing, eight states—Alabama, Georgia, Louisiana, Maine, Mississippi, Oklahoma, South Carolina, and Texas—have decided not to participate in the ACA. Five other states are leaning toward not participating. Of the remaining 37 states, 20 are undecided; 4 are leaning toward participating; 13 and the District of Columbia are moving forth with implementation.[1] Thus, the actual number of qualified individuals who will ultimately obtain insurance has been called into question.

In addition to expanding eligibility for Medicaid coverage to a larger group of people based on income, the expansion will extend coverage to people up to 138% of the federal poverty level, which is about $15,400 for a single individual and about $30,000 for a family of four. The ACA will also cover previously excluded groups such as low-income adults without children. Further, the law also requires individuals with incomes over 138% and below 400% of the federal poverty level to purchase insurance through state health insurance exchanges. A health insurance exchange is a set of state-regulated and standardized health care plans in the United States, from which individuals may purchase health insurance eligible for federal subsidies. All exchanges must be fully certified and operational by January 1, 2014, under federal law.[2] States may elect not to establish their own exchanges, may band together with other states to create an exchange, or may use a federal exchange program through which individuals will purchase insurance. The deadline for states to elect whether or not to establish their own exchanges was fast approaching at the time of this writing, and the exchanges must be operational by January 1, 2014.

## ESSENTIAL HEALTH BENEFITS

To provide structure for states in developing the basic benefit for exchanges, as well as for Medicaid expansion, the federal government established a minimum set of benefits that states must include. These benefits (called essential health benefits [EHBs]) include the following:

- Ambulatory patient services;
- Emergency services;
- Hospitalization;
- Maternity and newborn care;

- Mental health and substance use disorder (SUD) services, including behavioral health treatment;
- Prescription drugs;
- Rehabilitative and habilitative services and devices;
- Laboratory services;
- Preventive and wellness services and chronic disease management;
- Pediatric services, including oral and vision care.

In addition to these essential benefits, states will also select a benchmark plan to use as a model for establishing the benefits and services that will meet the needs of its citizens. States will be able to modify benefits under the benchmark plan as long as the value of coverage is not reduced.[3]

With the advent of the ACA, a clear change for many behavioral health consumers and families is that coverage will be available to millions more people with these concerns than ever before. Adults without children will be eligible for coverage through Medicaid or exchanges who have not been covered before. This has significant implications for not only the behavioral health issues for these people, but also for their physical health. As we know from a National Association of State Mental Health Program Directors (NASMHPD) study (Shea & Shern, 2011), consumers with mental illnesses are likely to die 20 to 25 years earlier than the general population. This is due not only to the effects of many psychoactive medications on the health of people, but also to lack of access to primary physical health care and prevention activities that can reduce or slow the onset or progression of physical health ailments.

## FURTHER PROVISIONS OF THE ACA

The ACA includes several other provisions with implications for the health of consumers and their families. Many behavioral health disorders often emerge in the teenage years and early adulthood. In the past, these young people were dropped from their parents' insurance coverage on reaching the age of 18 or ceasing to be full-time students. Now, in a portion of the ACA that has already been implemented, young people under the age of 26 can be included in their family's health insurance policy. In addition, exclusion of individuals from insurance coverage based on preexisting conditions has been eliminated, a change that has already taken place for those under age 19, and will be extended to all ages in January 2014.

Further requirements of the ACA include the elimination of annual and lifetime limits on insurance coverage. For individuals with chronic or long-term disorders such as schizophrenia or bipolar disorders, this is a major change. Families will not be as likely to face financial devastation in providing care to their family members with these disorders.

As the ACA is being implemented, the requirements and rules of the Paul Wellstone and Pete Domenici Mental Health Parity and Addiction Equity Act of 2008 (MHPAEA) are being completed. This act generally prevents group health plans and health insurance issuers that provide mental health and substance use disorder (MH/SUD) benefits from imposing less favorable benefit limitations than on medical or surgical coverage. Although the MHPAEA does not require that MH/SUD disorders be covered by insurance plans, the Act does call for equity of coverage when MH/SUD benefits are provided.[4]

The ACA, which includes requirements for parity for mental health and addiction services, provides opportunity for individuals with mental or substance use disorders. More individuals will be eligible for, and receive, health care insurance. Insurance will need to cover behavioral health services the same as it covers medical and surgical care. There is opportunity to assure that behavioral health care follows the guidelines and principles of a "good and modern" addiction and mental health service system. The ACA treats psychiatric illness like any other and removes obstacles to fair and rational treatment and provides a framework for integrating primary and behavioral health care.

The ACA also provides support for states to develop and fund health homes. According to the Henry J. Kaiser Family Foundation, health homes are "person-centered systems of care that facilitate access to and coordination of the full array of primary and acute physical health services, behavioral health care, and long-term community-based services and supports."[5] Care is expedited through the use of registries, information technology, health information exchange, and other processes that help assure individuals obtain needed care when and where they need it. Health homes seek to provide care in a culturally and linguistically appropriate manner.

In a review specifically focused on implications of the ACA on substance use services, Buck (2011) reminded readers that existing substance abuse treatments were different from other types of medical care in several ways, with treatment for SUDs often based in rehabilitation facilities rather than in hospital or clinic-based settings (Abrams, 2012). In addition, whereas professionals in medical and other clinics often have professional degrees in medicine or psychology, SUD treatment professionals often have limited training, often a bachelor's degree or less, and many have risen to their positions through a peer training process. Buck's (2011) review also described several other provisions of the ACA, including references to medical homes "designed to increase health service delivery through various types of integrated systems, often based on primary care including the integration of substance abuse and mental health services in general medical care" (p. 1404). The review also referred to several studies that suggest that a large infusion of funds through the ACA for federally qualified health centers (FQHCs) will increase the service capacities of these centers to 44 million persons by 2015, up from 18.8 million in 2009. Many of these new cases will have high levels of persons with behavioral health morbidity. Other trends anticipated are declines in block grant money for SUD treatment efforts or other forms of therapy, and increases in the pressure to overemphasize traditional biological aspects of SUD treatment regimes or other forms of therapy along with a caution that essential benefits definitions across programs might not always include the full array of SUD coverage desired, especially in the social support domains (Abrams, 2012).

Health homes and other measures to assure coordination of primary care and behavioral health care will be enhanced with another initiative included in the ACA: support for development of electronic health records. Electronic health records offer support for coordination of health care. With sufficient protections for concerns of confidentiality, health care providers and recipients of behavioral health services will be able to coordinate an individual's care.

Additional technologies, such as telemedicine, will enable access to care in rural and frontier communities where it might otherwise be unavailable. Telemedicine enables specialists to interact with health care providers and recipients of care regardless of location. This is especially important in specialty fields where there is a shortage in the workforce, such as psychiatry. Telemedicine is also being used in conjunction with the medical home model, allowing persons under care to communicate with their treatment professionals from their own homes, and facilitating communication among various professionals involved in patient care.

## FOCUS ON RECOVERY

Of great importance to behavioral health consumers and their families is that the ACA continues to move forward the progress made over the last decades in moving the treatment system to a more person-centered recovery model from a medically driven "maintenance" model that has been challenging, yet rewarding. The medically driven model has an emphasis on illness and symptoms, whereas the recovery model is about thriving instead of merely surviving. The recovery model values self-direction, recognizing individuals' needs and desires in regard to their health care. The recovery model allows individuals, not a medical textbook, to define their own recovery. Shared decision making is a strategy that fosters recovery, and encourages individuals to be more active participants in their health care. The ACA supports and promotes person-centered care and shared decision making (SDM) in efforts to improve quality of care. SDM includes recipient and provider communication and decision-making tools. SDM tools allow the health care provider and the individual to open a dialogue about health issues, and help individuals make informed choices about their health care. Individuals

THE AFFORDABLE CARE ACT AND INTEGRATED BEHAVIORAL HEALTH CARE

who are engaged in their health care planning can experience much better outcomes because they have worked with their health care provider to set their own goals. It balances clinical information with an individual's preferences, goals, cultural values, and beliefs. Many health care providers have developed libraries of DVDs and print materials to assist individuals in participating in decisions for their health care. In the behavioral health sector, the Substance Abuse and Mental Health Services Administration (SAMHSA) has provided tools to assist recipients of mental health services in the process of person-centered care and SDM.[6]

The United States currently dedicates only 3% of its health care budget to disease prevention and public health. The ACA makes it easier for individuals to access preventive services, and addresses this disparity through the creation of the National Prevention, Health Promotion and Public Health Council, which will coordinate and execute a comprehensive strategy; and the Prevention and Public Health Fund, which will invest in prevention and public health programs to improve health and reduce health costs. Cancer screenings, vaccinations, tobacco cessation, and other prevention services in many cases will be provided free of charge under the law. The term *prevention* is common in the substance abuse and addiction field. There are prevention strategies in communities that address alcohol, tobacco, and other substances. It has been estimated that investments in prevention programs that encourage physical activity, good nutrition, and tobacco cessation can yield excellent returns on the investment, returning an overall $5.60 in health cost savings for every $1 spent (Trust for America's Health, 2008).

Prevention is not as common a term in the mental health community. We seem to struggle with the idea that mental illness can be prevented. Mental illness can be triggered by external trauma, as well as biological factors. If individuals have appropriate coping skills to deal with trauma as it arises, they can reduce the chances that a mental health crisis will happen. Developing a plan to raise awareness of one's current coping skills, and a plan for addressing potential triggers, can be a prevention strategy for maintaining mental health and wellness.

By including mental health and SUD services as mandated services, the ACA is moving us closer to the realization that one's mind and body are connected, and integrating mental health and physical health together is beneficial. A more holistic approach will improve health outcomes and engage individuals in healthy dialogues with their practitioners. A recovery-driven, integrated approach to health care can reduce the stigma associated with seeking behavioral health services, and will encourage individuals to accept responsibility for their own recovery.

The ACA also makes it easier for individuals who might need long-term care to receive that care in their own home instead of a facility. This is accomplished through giving states more flexibility in their Medicaid plans. Before the ACA, statutes limited the number of services that could be included as a benefit under Home and Community Based Services. The ACA removes the limitation on Center for Medicare and Medicaid Services (CMS) authority and allows states to include, subject to CMS approval, additional services beyond the ones specifically identified in the statute. Removing this barrier will keep many older individuals with physical health challenges who might have a cooccurring behavioral health issue in the community and give them access to needed care.

Workforce issues always impact the availability and the quality of our health care. With an increased focus on integration of health care, a more diverse workforce is needed. There must be a health care workforce that is more knowledgeable of behavioral health and physical health issues, and that can work as a team to engage the individual in a meaningful health care relationship. The ACA is an opportunity to bridge the historically separated systems of primary care and behavioral health by integrating services. One such opportunity is to employ individuals with behavioral health needs as health and wellness coaches. Individuals who have a background in peer support as a peer support specialist, or as an addiction recovery coach can be trained as health and wellness coaches within FQHCs and other health care settings. Using their peer support skills, along with their life experiences with behavioral health challenges, peers can engage other peers in conversations about health and wellness and establish a meaningful mutual relationship that can also benefit the other health care providers on the team.

## WHAT PLANNING COUNCILS CAN DO

As the ACA is implemented, behavioral health consumers, family members, and interested stakeholders must remain vigilant and active in the state and federal planning processes. Because many people are not familiar with the ACA, consumers and family members can educate themselves about the Act and share that knowledge with others. One way to do that is for consumers and family members to get involved with the Mental Health Planning and Advisory Council (PAC) in their state. These PACs exist in every state and territory as a condition of receiving federal mental health block grant funds. Although the PACs might go by different names in various states, including the more recent term Behavioral Health Planning Council, the state agency that oversees mental health services will be able to provide information about how to contact the PAC.

PACs are in a unique position to impact the implementation of the ACA and assure appropriate application of EHBs. Every state and territory has a PAC as a condition to receive the Community Mental Health Services Block Grant (Pub. L. 106-310). The law specifies required membership and outlines the purposes of the PAC.

Councils must include representatives from several state agencies and representatives of public and private entities concerned with the need, planning, operation, funding, and use of mental health services and related support services. PACs must also include adults with serious mental illness who are receiving or have received mental health services and families of such adults, as well as families of children with serious emotional disturbance. Not less than 50% of the members must be individuals who are not state employees or providers of mental health services. In addition to these membership requirements, some PACs have elected to assure representation of diverse ethnic and linguistic communities; youth; older adults; individuals from the lesbian, bisexual, gay, transgender, and questioning communities; veterans; faith-based and advocacy organizations, and state agencies.

Members of PACs who are not state employees or providers of services are not only recipients or former recipients of services or family members of recipients or members of the PAC. These individuals also belong to organizations like a consumer association, the National Alliance on Mental Illness, United States Psychiatric Rehabilitation Association, National Council for Community Behavioral Healthcare, Mental Health America, and Protection Advocacy for Mental Illness Advisory Councils.

The required purposes of the PAC are (a) to assist the Mental Health Authority in the development of the state plan and application for the Community Mental Health Services Block Grant; (b) to monitor, review, and evaluate the allocation and adequacy of mental health services in the state; and (c) to serve as advocates for adults with serious mental illness, children with a serious emotional disturbance, and other individuals with mental illnesses or emotional problems.

These required purposes are broad to enable and encourage PACs to undertake activities relevant to behavioral health issues in their state. For example, some PACs assist in developing assessments of behavioral health needs and creating the mental health plan for the block grants; others establish processes to review and comment on the plan and application before it is submitted to SAMHSA. Some PACs conduct on-site reviews of behavioral health services; others rely on a review of outcome data produced by the state. Some PACs have very strong relationships with legislators who might determine the future of publicly funded behavioral health services; others rely on white papers and public education to advocate for behavioral health services.

In addition to membership requirements and mandated purposes, PACs often span tenures of governors, mental health commissioners, or directors of the single state authority for substance abuse prevention and treatment; the PAC agenda continues regardless of changes in government. State agencies required to be members of the PAC might also change leadership, but the voices of recipients and families of recipients continue through changes in governmental leadership.

Starting with Fiscal Year 2011, SAMHSA permitted states to submit a combined application for the Community Mental Health Services Block Grant and the Substance Abuse Prevention and Treatment Block Grant. Announcements for the combined application process included an "encouragement" that PACs consider expanding their focus to include substance abuse prevention and treatment issues.

In an effort to understand how PACs nationwide are addressing this expansion issue, the West Virginia Mental Health Planning Council (WVMHPC) conducted a national survey of PACs and state mental health planners in 2012 to determine if PACs were including substance abuse issues and if current or former recipients of substance abuse treatment services, substance abuse prevention and treatment service representatives, or both were members of PACs. Representatives from nearly half the states and territories responded. Although 40% of the respondents indicated the existence of a separate planning or advisory council for substance abuse in their state, 70% reported the PAC included individuals in recovery from substance abuse and a like number reported the single state authority for substance abuse was represented. Many PACs have been integrated for several years.

One respondent wrote concerning an integrated Council, "Members now have a more systems framework of thinking, understanding how it all ties in together. There is a good balance of discussion and debate about issues . . . everyone can hear and see the other side that they may not be familiar with. . . . Empathy has grown amongst the group." Another comment was, "We are about the mission of helping people rather than separate illnesses."

"Integrating substance abuse prevention and treatment into the Mental Health Planning and Advisory Council has led to forging new partnerships among both state agencies/divisions and service providers," indicated one respondent. Another wrote, "It allows for a widening of the circle and a bigger arena for reviewing policy, identifying gaps, making recommendations, etc. It allows for making better decisions about integrated treatment for co-occurring disorders."

The diversity of membership of PACs provides the opportunity to impact implementation of the ACA, particularly regarding the establishment of the EHB and assurance of parity for mental illness (including substance abuse). People who have received or are receiving treatment for a mental illness or substance abuse know what works. Families of people who have received or are receiving treatment know what works. It will be essential for these voices to review and comment on proposed EHBs to assure that effective approaches to treatment are included.

Following adoption of the EHB and implementation of health insurance coverage to meet the requirements of the ACA, PACs are in a position to monitor and evaluate the effectiveness of implementation. Many PACs have experience in monitoring and evaluating the effectiveness of mental health and substance abuse services in their role with block grants and other publicly funded behavioral health services.

For example, in West Virginia, current and former recipients of mental health services and family members of recipients who were members of the Planning Council voiced concerns over the responsiveness and effectiveness of crisis intervention services throughout the state. The WVMHPC undertook a two-pronged approach to identify issues beyond anecdotes. The first was to develop a "secret shopper" approach, using scripted telephone calls to crisis lines, identifying a crisis, and seeking assistance. Volunteers then reported the outcome of those contacts: the time it took for the call to be answered, the qualifications of the respondent, and the level of helpfulness of the respondent. The second approach was to conduct interviews with key staff of each primary provider of mental health services to determine that provider's policies concerning crisis intervention, comparing them with the Mental Health Authority's requirements. The outcomes of these activities were reported with recommendations to providers and the Mental Health Authority for systemic improvements.

In another activity, the WVMHPC undertook to compare West Virginia's mental health system with the goals of the President's New Freedom Commission on Mental Health and offered recommendations to achieve more congruence.

PACs could use either of these approaches to monitor and evaluate the effectiveness of implementing EHBs as they address the needs of individuals with mental health or SUDs.

States will have options to design insurance exchanges, modify or expand Medicaid, and undertake other revisions to implement the ACA. The first role of the PAC will be to become aware of and understand which of these options the state is choosing. During this process, the PAC will want to be assured that parity is being addressed—that treatment limitations applied to behavioral health are not more restrictive than those applied to medical and surgical care.

PACs will also want to assure that coverage is provided for a good and modern behavioral health care system. SAMHSA suggests that a good and modern mental health and addiction service system provides a continuum of effective treatment and support services that span health care, employment, housing, and educational sectors. Integration of primary care and behavioral health are essential. SAMHSA has identified the key elements of behavioral health services that should be provided.

Following the design of insurance exchanges and making decisions about Medicaid coverage, states will undertake enrolling individuals in the health insurance plans that will be available. PACs have a role in this activity, too. PACs should develop and implement information activities to inform potential and current recipients of behavioral health services of the available plans and options for enrollment in those plans. Some PACs are familiar with this type of outreach and education, having served to encourage enrollment in the Children's Health Insurance Program. PACs might want to adapt public education materials from Families USA, "The Voice for Health Care Consumers."[7] Families USA is an excellent resource for learning about the ACA and developing outreach and advocacy for quality health care, including behavioral health care.

Depending on the structure of the PAC, the organization might recruit volunteers to work with navigators or an in-person assistance program (IPAP), or they might apply to serve as an IPAP. Council members who are affiliated with a related nonprofit organization such as the National Alliance on Mental Illness (NAMI), Mental Health America, or a consumer-operated organization could encourage that organization to apply to be an IPAP. Navigators and IPAPs provide public education and assistance in enrolling in health insurance plans established by the state under the auspices of the ACA.

PACs could also develop public education and information activities to inform eligible individuals of the availability of Medicaid coverage. Many states will take advantage of new eligibility requirements and the federal participation for Medicaid; there will be 100% federal reimbursement for new enrollees for 3 years and no less than 90% thereafter. It is anticipated the new requirements for enrolling in Medicaid will greatly expand the number of persons with SUDs who will be eligible. MHPACs can use this opportunity to conduct outreach and information activities to this population. PACs are in a position to affect service system design, encourage enrollment, and monitor the implementation of the ACA as it affects individuals with behavioral health issues.

As the country moves forward in implementing the ACA, consumers and family members will be faced with the need to adapt to a rapidly evolving health care landscape. Along with the challenges of learning to enroll in new systems such as expanded Medicaid programs or health exchanges, exciting opportunities lie ahead for consumers and families. As the focus on recovery and self-directed care continues to grow, people will be able to be increasingly knowledgeable about, and in control of, their own medical care. Further, new technologies will improve the ways in which consumers communicate with treatment professionals, as well as improving coordination of care among treating professionals. Existing new technologies such as electronic health records and telemedicine are part of that change, along with new technologies, such as the use of social media and telephone-based applications to improve care and communication. Opportunities also exist for consumers and family members to be involved in ACA implementation by serving as peer providers or addiction recovery coaches in new models of care. Working collaboratively with state behavioral health planning councils or other state advocacy organizations, consumers and family members will also be instrumental in educating themselves and others about the

ACA and helping to expand enrollment to improve access to as broad a base as possible, as well as assisting the U.S. health care system to understand and accept behavioral health as being essential to health.

## NOTES

1. Dailybriefing@advisory.com.
2. http://www.informationweek.com/news/healthcare/policy/231001432.
3. http://www.healthcare.gov/news/factsheets/2011/12/essential-health-benefits12162011a.html.
4. http://cciio.cms.gov/programs/protections/mhpaea/mhpaea_factsheet.html.
5. http://www.kff.org/medicaid/upload/8136.pdf.
6. http://www.samhsa.gov/consumersurvivor/sdm/starthere.html.
7. http://www.familiesusa.org/.

## REFERENCES

Abrams, M. T. (2012). *Coordination of care for persons with substance use disorders under the Affordable Care Act: Opportunities and challenges.* Baltimore, MD: The Hilltop Institute, University of Maryland, Baltimore Campus.

Buck, J. A. (2011). The looming expansion and transformation of public substance abuse treatment under the Affordable Care Act. *Health Affairs (Millwood), 30,* 1402–1410.

Shea, P., & Shern, D. (2011). *Primary prevention in behavioral health: Investing in our nation's future.* Alexandria, VA: National Association of State Mental Health Program Directors.

Trust for America's Health. (2008). *Prevention for a healthier America: Investments in disease prevention yield significant savings, stronger communities.* Washington, DC: Author. Retrieved from www.healthyamericans.org

# Women's Health and Behavioral Health Issues in Health Care Reform

JEAN LAU CHIN

*Derner Institute for Advanced Psychological Studies, Adelphi University, Garden City, New York, USA*

BARBARA W. K. YEE

*Department of Family and Consumer Sciences, University of Hawaii at Manoa, Honolulu, Hawaii, USA*

MARTHA E. BANKS

*ABackans DCP, Inc., Akron, Ohio, USA*

*As health care reform promises to change the landscape of health care delivery, its potential impact on women's health looms large. Whereas health and mental health systems have historically been fragmented, the Affordable Care Act (ACA) mandates integrated health care as the strategy for reform. Current systems fragment women's health not only in their primary care, mental health, obstetrical, and gynecological needs, but also in their roles as the primary caregivers for parents, spouses, and children. Changes in reimbursement, and in restructuring financing and care coordination systems through accountable care organizations and medical homes, will potentially improve women's health care.*

The Affordable Care Act (ACA) is the single greatest legislative leap forward in history for people with substance abuse and mental health disorders. In a single act (albeit a complicated one), it sends the message that behavioral health is integral to health. It provides various mechanisms that encourage an integrated approach to health care that includes as much behavioral health care as a person needs. With integration, however, comes personal responsibility, a healing concept for those in recovery, but a difficult endeavor for those most seriously compromised by their illnesses (Emmet, Morgan, & Stange, this issue).

The ACA encourages early intervention, encourages greater awareness of behavioral health in primary care, and offers prevention incentives. As health care reform promises to change the landscape of how access to and utilization of care will occur, it is important to look at its impact on women as a population of interest, and the integration of health care as the strategy for how reform will occur. Historically, health and mental health systems of care have been parallel silos. The systems were designed with separate doors of entry for reimbursement, access, and utilization. Communications between physicians and mental health professionals were met by a solid wall presumably based on the specialization within health care. The ACA created a mandate for integrated health care. As we begin to incorporate holistic concepts of health and health care, we find that the historical systems of care promoted fragmented care, which has had particular implications for women. We find bias in its inattention to the special needs of women and the particular burdens they bear. Women make the majority of health care decisions, on average live longer than men, and require more medical care over a longer period of time. They are often the primary caregivers for parents and children. These roles become magnified when they themselves have physical or mental disabilities, encounter major illness, or simply need to cope with developmental tasks of reproduction, childbearing, menopause, and aging. Stress and coping mechanisms might well increase the prevalence of depression and anxiety. How will health care reform help or hinder the care for women's health? Elements of the ACA, including changes in reimbursement, availability of insurance coverage, accountable care organizations, medical homes, and health technology, are but a few of the more important challenges facing women as they negotiate a new system of care delivery under health care reform.

As Manderscheid (this issue) suggests, the ACA holds promise to improve the future of behavioral health care through transforming our broader insurance and care delivery systems. He summarizes key features of the ACA, which include (a) mental health parity in the ACA as a floor benefit, and (b) reform at five levels (i.e., insurance, coverage, quality, performance, and information technology). The ACA will be implemented in an environment of rapid change that includes moving toward an integrated system of care, and addressing social justice concerns regarding health status and health care. Social justice demands that we value all people equally. Thus, we need to address these class-related health disparities by promoting equity in health status and care. A major focus of the ACA is to promote equity in health insurance coverage and access to care to reduce health disparities.

Given these foci of the ACA, how do women fare? Families USA (2012) believes that "Being a Woman Just Got a Little Easier" as far as how the ACA benefits women. Historically, women have not had equal access to essential health coverage and care. They have been charged higher insurance premiums than men simply because they were women—that is, they were considered a higher risk group. Even then, there was no guarantee that the health coverage they purchased would cover the women's health services that they needed. The ACA promises to change that; the law improves access to care that is essential to women's health and makes coverage more affordable. Families USA (2012) developed a fact sheet outlining key elements of the ACA for women. These include the following:

- Women can now visit an OB-GYN without a referral or prior approval; under the old system, it was considered specialty care.
- Pregnant women who have Medicaid now have more options for where they get their maternity care. They can choose to get care at a free-standing birth center, for example.
- Women can now obtain preventive services with no copays or deductibles. This includes mammograms, cervical cancer screenings, and blood pressure screenings. New health plans must cover additional preventive services for women with no copays or deductibles. These include:
  - An annual well woman visit.
  - Birth control, including oral contraception and intrauterine devices.
  - HIV screening and counseling.
  - Sexually transmitted infection counseling.
  - Screening for gestational diabetes.
  - Breastfeeding consultation and supplies, including breast pumps.
  - Screening and counseling for domestic violence.
  - Starting in 2014, health plans will have to include coverage for maternity services.

## ADDRESSING BARRIERS TO CARE

### Cost Is No Longer a Barrier to Preventive Care

Although every woman should be able to obtain the preventive health care services she needs, many women in the past have had to forgo lifesaving and cost-effective preventive care because of cost. Today, birth control costs women with health insurance about, $215 a year. Women who are uninsured currently have to pay even more to obtain birth control, about $1,210 a year. Breast pumps and accessories can cost new moms about $300 to $750 each year. Starting in August 2013, new health plans are required to cover these supplies with no copays.

However, some women still lack knowledge about contraceptives. A survey by Teva Women's Health, which manufactures contraceptives, found that two in five women said that they did not use contraception or skipped doses of birth control pills, mostly because they were not sexually active at the time or believed they were infertile (AFP-Relaxnews, 2012). In addition, there are many who oppose the use of contraceptives. Michael New of the antiabortion research organization the Charlotte Lozier Institute, said that antiabortion rights legislation should be designed to increase "the costs" of the procedure to discourage women from obtaining abortions. The biggest contraceptive controversy emerged during a House committee hearing on the proposed Blunt amendment to the ACA to consider whether religious freedom trumps contraception coverage, which discounted Georgetown third-year law student Sandra Fluke as an "unqualified" witness, leaving only men to testify during the first panel. House Minority Leader Nancy Pelosi (D-CA), countered with an unofficial hearing on women's health solely featuring Fluke, who spoke about a gay female friend who could not afford birth control pills to control a cyst and ended up in the emergency room to remove her ovaries. Radio host Rush Limbaugh then declared that Fluke was "a slut . . . a prostitute. She wants to be paid to have sex," and that all "feminazis" should post sex videos online in exchange for taxpayer-subsidized birth control (Chan, 2012).

## Costs of Health Insurance

Other provisions of the ACA will extend health coverage. Young adults can now remain on their parents' health plan up to the age of 26. More than 3 million young adults have already gained coverage under this provision of the law. Low- and middle-income families will receive tax credits to help make coverage affordable. This means that 7 million women who are currently uninsured will be able to get tax credits that cover a portion of their monthly health insurance premiums, making coverage more affordable for them and their families. More low-income adults will be eligible for Medicaid; about 10 million women who are currently uninsured might be able to get health coverage through Medicaid. The law also provides greater health care security for women and their families and makes coverage more affordable.

## Being a Woman Will No Longer Be a Preexisting Condition

As Nancy Pelosi, House Speaker, said, "If you are a woman, if you are in child-bearing age and you have children, it's a preexisting condition. If you can't have children, it's a preexisting condition. If you have a C-section, it's a preexisting condition. If you are a victim of domestic abuse, it is a preexisting condition" (Goudreau, 2010). In the past, this has been the way in which health insurance companies had a number of provisions to deny coverage. This can no longer happen under the ACA.

Health insurance companies can no longer deny children health coverage because they have a preexisting condition or deny children coverage for health services to treat their preexisting condition as they have done in the past. They can no longer cancel your health coverage when you get sick. They can no longer place lifetime dollar limits on your coverage. They will no longer be able to deny anyone health coverage or charge more for health coverage based on a preexisting condition.

Nearly 30% of women (28.4%) in the United States have a diagnosed preexisting condition that, without the health care law, could lead to a denial of coverage. Now they also will not be denied coverage for having had a C-section or for having been a victim of domestic violence.

Insurance companies will no longer be able to charge women higher premiums than men for the exact same health coverage. This will ensure that no woman is ever again charged up to 85% more than a man for the exact same health coverage, simply because she is a woman. It ends discrimination against women by insurance companies.

The ACA recognizes the specific needs of women and mothers. Employers must now provide nursing mothers with breaks and a private space to express breast milk in the workplace. This protects 19 million employed women and ensures that working moms can make the personal decision whether or not to breastfeed without worrying about potential negative consequences at their jobs. Provisions are being made by states to provide comprehensive and evidence-based sex education. This will help to reduce teen pregnancy rates and the transmission of sexually transmitted infections. Already more than $100 million in grants have been awarded to states to provide youth with comprehensive sex education programs.

## MEDICAL HEALTH HOMES

The principal tool envisioned by the ACA to improve the quality of health care is the health home. The mechanism to foster the development of a health home is an accountable care organization (ACO). Although this mechanism is a work in progress, health homes are intended to integrate behavioral and primary care so that all of a person's health needs can be addressed through a single entity. They also offer disease prevention and health promotion interventions. Typically, they are responsible for the health care of a defined population. ACOs, on the other hand, represent the organizational arrangements put in place to operate health homes. An ACO can be a lead organization that coordinates the activities of several subsidiary organizations, or it can be an entire new entity created specifically to operate a health home. In either case, it represents a new organizational arrangement for delivering coordinated health care (Manderscheid, this issue). These medical health homes will be financed by moving Medicaid and Medicare financing systems toward annual case rates (per person served) or annual capitation rates (per person covered), hence combining both financing systems with systems to manage financing that have the potential to replace traditional managed care.

What is unclear is how behavioral health will be integrated into the medical health home; in fact, proposals are underway for behavioral health homes to integrate mental health, substance abuse, and health because conditions often are cooccurring (Croghan & Brown, 2010). How can or will these medical health homes benefit women? Integrated health care has potential for providing a seamless continuum of care for women across their life spans that links wellness with prenatal care and family planning to medical care. The medical home concept has potential for improving patient choice, affordability, and access, and in being accountable to women and their specific needs. It could promote reimbursement mechanisms that would reflect care coordination, cost savings, and interdisciplinary practice.

## CONTRACEPTION AND REPRODUCTIVE CARE

Issues of contraception and reproductive care, a primary concern and role among women, raise many issues in addition to costs. It is unclear how this will play out in the ACA. There continues to be major disagreement over the issue of coverage for contraception and abortions related to religious and moral opinions about pro-choice versus pro-life that deter rapid settlement. Attitudes prevail about women and women's sexuality that could also pose barriers to change. In a recent statement that was both factually inaccurate and horribly offensive, Republican Missouri Senate candidate Rep. Todd Akin (Moore, 2012) said that victims of "legitimate rape" do not get pregnant because "the female body has ways to try to shut that whole thing down." Mitt Romney and Paul Ryan tried to distance themselves from the remark, although they were in lockstep with Akin on the major women's health issues of our time. The Republican Party voted to include the "Human Life Amendment" in their platform, calling for a constitutional ban on abortions nationwide, even for rape victims (Shen, 2012).

Akin's faux pas is troubling for what it suggests regarding women and sex (Goodwin, 2012). Implicitly, the comment conveys that only consensual sex results in pregnancy—and not incest, marital rape, war rape, date rape, and other types of sexual coercion and abuse. Among American cases of known rape pregnancies involving adolescents, a majority of victims are biologically related to their perpetrators. Nearly a third of the rape victims "did not discover they were pregnant until they had already entered the second trimester." The researchers discovered that less than 12% of the pregnancies resulted in a spontaneous abortion. The authors concluded that sexual victimization "frequently" leads to unwanted pregnancies. Akin's comment illuminates how a predominantly male electorate is shaping the political and regulatory discourse on women's reproduction. For example, a range of fetal-protection laws are now implemented and variously enforced in 37 states. Many of the laws are overly broad and unusually vague, criminalizing any and all activities that could harm a fetus. Most of these efforts ultimately target pregnant women.

It is particularly ironic that TRICARE—the military's health insurance plan—"denies coverage for abortions for rape and incest, given the long-standing challenges the armed services have faced in addressing sexual assault among the ranks" (Korb & Arons, 2012).

## WOMEN: OVERWHELMING CAREGIVING BURDENS AFFECT HEALTH CARE

The ACA will provide needed relief for the tremendous stress and strains of caregiving burdens that are disproportionately shouldered by women, ethnic minorities, and low-income families around the globe (Braun, Yee, Brown, & Mokuau, 2004; Yee, DeBaryshe, Yuen, Kim, & McCubbin, 2006). An analysis by the National Alliance for Caregiving in collaboration with AARP (2009) found that females provide about 66% of the care for recipients who are older and female. Eighty-six percent of caregivers were related to care recipients, with 36% taking care of a parent. Older caregivers are likely to be sole unpaid caregivers without the support of other unpaid caregivers at 47%, in comparison to younger caregivers at 30%. These older caregivers, older than 65, are likely to be wives or siblings of the recipient of that care.

Ethnicity of caregivers mediates the nature of the caregiving relationship. For example, the National Alliance for Caregiving and AARP (2009) found that Hispanic caregivers are younger than White or African American caregivers, and Hispanic and Asian caregivers are less likely to be married than White caregivers. This latter finding might be related to immigration patterns for Hispanic and Asian populations in which parents of immigrants are less likely to be in the United States than White or African American populations. This pattern occurs among more recent immigrants, rather than for ethnic minority populations who have been living in the United States for three or more generations, such as Asians who settled in Hawaii prior to the 1950s.

In a recent study, Yancura (2013) found that culture makes an impact on the justifications for caregiving among White, Asian American, and Native Hawaiian grandparents raising grandchildren. She found that Native Hawaiian grandparents had the highest level of custom justification (i.e., cultural expectation for grandparents to be stewards of Hawaiian cultural values in families) of providing care to their grandchildren, Asian American grandparents were in the middle, and White grandparents the least, using a custom justification. In contrast, Native Hawaiian grandparents scored higher than Asian American grandparents in felt responsibility (i.e., duty to one's family) for their grandchildren, but were nonsignificantly distinct to White grandparents.

The MetLife Mature Market Institute's (2011) study of parent caregiving and its impact among baby boomers suggested that this family caregiving has tripled in the last 15 years and about 25% of adult children provide care to their parents. The financial parent caregiving burden in aggregated lost wages is approximately $324,044 for women (*i.e.*, $142,693 in lost wages, $50,000 in pension losses, and $142,693 in lost Social Security benefits). Women provide basic care and those adult children caregivers are more likely to have fair or poor health than those who do not provide care to their parents. Family caregiving is likely to have increased the burden in families with limited English proficiency (Sanchez, Chapa, Ybarra, & Martinez, 2012). The negative financial impacts and poorer health outcomes for women caregivers are a great sacrifice with serious and negative consequences for the caregivers' personal welfare.

Caregivers not only face additional financial burdens, but there could be negative health and mental health consequences for that family's sacrifice and service (National Alliance for Caregiving in collaboration with AARP, 2009). For example, caretakers typically have lower family incomes and high coresidence rates, creating greater stress and strain associated with the caregiving. The greater the length of care, 5 years or more, the greater the reported negative self-report of fair or poor health as a consequence of that caregiving. Thirty-one percent of caregivers report that caregiving is emotionally stressful and leads to less time with other family members.

Caregiving burdens exact a huge toll on those providing care when caregiving is lengthy (National Alliance for Caregiving, 2011) and intense, such as those providing care for family members with Alzheimer's disease. According to the REACH1 project (Resources for Enhancing Alzheimer's Caregiver Health), as care recipients' health declined steadily in such areas as cognitive abilities and the need for assistance on activities of daily living, caregivers were likely to show increases in depression and use of medical services (Kim, Chang, Rose, & Kim, 2011). These authors found that the extent of caregiver burdens were predicted by the extent of disease-related factors such as greater impairments in activities of daily living and instrumental activities of daily living. Higher caregiver burdens were reported to a greater extent by older, female, spousal relationships, and coresidence with the care recipient. Those who used a greater number of coping strategies had higher levels of caregiving burden. This latter finding must be explored to understand whether caregivers used a greater number of coping strategies to alleviate high caregiver burdens, or whether the caregiver tried many ineffective coping strategies earlier in the process, and when they did not work, tried additional ones to see if they would help to alleviate the stress and strain of high caregiver burdens.

The ACA promotes the central importance of person- and family-centered care in the design and delivery of new models of care to improve quality and efficiency of health care, including assessment of family caregivers' experience of care. Coupled with the National Family Caregiver Support Program under the Older American Act in 2000, family caregivers are considered consumers; the program provides grants to states to fund services and supports that assist family and friends in caring for their loved ones at home. This will help relieve the great caregiving burden on families, and especially women (Feinberg, Reinhard, Houser, & Chula, 2011). Allowing spouses to be paid by Medicaid for personal care services has not had a negative impact on older patient outcomes (Newcomer, Kang, & Doty, 2011).

The ACA will enhance the opportunities to address some of the negative health outcomes for older people and their caregivers. For example, Dong, Chang, Wong, and Simon (2012) found that Chinese elders exhibited more depressive symptoms than other elders with feelings of helplessness, dissatisfaction with life, feelings of boredom and loss of interest in activities, suicidal ideation, and worthlessness. These depressive symptoms were associated with societal and family conflicts, financial constraints, and the worsening of their physical health.

## WOMEN WITH DISABILITIES

An overview of health care issues faced by women with disabilities warrants consideration with reference to specific sections of the ACA to address their special issues. The literature is sparse addressing health care for women with disabilities; information about health care disparities is largely extrapolated from information about gender and ethnicity without regard to ability status. Women with disabilities face greater challenges in accessing health care because they are often considered to have preexisting conditions; their greater difficulty in finding affordable health insurance and receiving health care have been empirically supported. Often their health care is limited to their specific disabilities, and they are often not assessed for victimization.

It is important to understand what is meant by disability. Section 902 of the Americans with Disabilities Act (ADA, 2008) defines disability as:

1. a physical or mental impairment that substantially limits one or more of the major life activities of such individual;
2. a record of such an impairment; or
3. being regarded as having such an impairment. (p. 1)

Furthermore, Borneman (2009) observed, "Mental health and physical health are as inextricably linked as their counterparts, mental illness and physical illness. The latter can result in various short- and long-term disabilities" (p. ix). Women with disabilities benefit from several of the provisions of the ACA.

## Preexisting Conditions

Perhaps the most obvious issue is concern about preexisting conditions that have historically been used to deny insurance coverage to women with disabilities. Jarrett, Yee, and Banks (2007) identified lack of health insurance as contributing to "premature death, disease, and disability" (p. 311) for women.

Banks (2013) described a broad range of disabling conditions experienced by women, noting that some are congenital whereas others are acquired.

> In the case of acquired disabilities, usually an initial medical response involves seeking a "cure" or removal of the disabling condition in order to bring a person "back to normal." In some cases, disabilities can be acute, such as in the case of a broken bone that heals with or without treatment, after which the person with a disability is able to resume previous activities. In other situations, a chronic or ongoing disabling condition, such as paralysis following a severe stroke, does not respond or only responds partially to treatment. In such cases, the treatment focus moves away from "cure" and toward compensation and accommodation. Some disabling conditions, such as Alzheimer's dementia are progressive. While there might be a slowing of the condition with treatment, the downward progression does not stop (p. 467).

The broad range of disability requires a variety of treatments and a clear understanding that women with disabilities must be assessed individually to receive appropriate health care. For disabling conditions expected to last until the end of a woman's life, critical parts of the ACA are Section 2711 (No Lifetime or Annual Limits) and Section 2712 (Prohibition on Rescissions; Patient Protection and Affordable Care Act, 2010).

Given the discrimination noted earlier against all women by health insurance companies, it can be expected that women with disabilities who had disabilities prior to applying for insurance would have had minimal opportunities to obtain needed insurance. Section 1101 (Immediate Access to Insurance for Uninsured Individuals With a Preexisting Condition of the Affordable Care Act; Patient Protection and Affordable Care Act, 2010) makes such discrimination illegal and establishes "a temporary high risk health insurance pool program to provide health insurance coverage" (p. 45) until January 1, 2014, to give insurance companies time to comply. Section 2704 (Prohibition of Preexisting Condition Exclusions or Other Discrimination Based on Health Status) and Section 2705 (Prohibiting Discrimination Against Individual Participants and Beneficiaries Based on Health Status) provide additional support for access to health care insurance for women with disabilities.

## Finding and Affording Health Insurance

The ADA applies to all businesses with 15 or more employees. Small businesses, which employ people with disabilities at significantly higher rates than big businesses (Kaye, 2003), struggle with costs of accommodations for people with disabilities, including the cost of health insurance. Businesses with 15 to 100 employees are provided with support through Section 1311 of the ACA to afford health insurance for all employees, including women with disabilities. Section 1311 describes Small Business Health Options Programs that are to be fully instituted by January 1, 2014. The ability of individual consumers and employers to find affordable health insurance should facilitate the obtaining of health care for women with disabilities and hopefully, enhance the employment possibilities for women with disabilities.

Many women with disabilities live in poverty (American Psychological Association, 2007; Banks & Marshall, 2004). For this reason, it is critical that health care be affordable. Section 1103 of the Affordable Care Act (Patient Protection and Affordable Care Act, 2010) creates access to information so that consumers can identify and compare general insurance coverage options. It should be noted that there is a specific exclusion of "other than coverage that provides reimbursement only for the treatment or mitigation of—(i) a single disease or condition; or (ii) an unreasonably limited set of diseases or conditions" (pp. 58–59); such insurance might be of particular interest to women with disabilities, especially for disabling conditions that disproportionately affect women, such as multiple sclerosis. As the ACA is implemented, it will be important to consider ways to include access to specialized health insurance.

## Assessment for Victimization

Women with disabilities, on average, endure domestic violence for longer periods than women without disabilities and are at high risk for being abused by multiple perpetrators (Banks, 2007). In addition to the emotional, physical, and sexual abuse generally considered as manifestations of domestic violence, Nosek, Foley, Hughes, and Howland (2001) found that women with disabilities described five types of domestic violence:

1. Disability-related emotional abuse,
2. Disability-related physical abuse,
3. Disability-related sexual abuse,
4. Abuse related to disability-related settings, and
5. Abuse related to helping relationships. (p. 182)

Therefore, it is critical that health care include assessment for abuse. There are provisions in the ACA addressing the need for assessment of and determination of risk for domestic violence for pregnant adolescents and women, but specific attention is given to assessment and risks for women with disabilities.

## Comprehensive Health Care: Focus on the Whole Woman, Not Just the Identified Disability

Banks (2010) noted, "Women with disabilities seldom receive comprehensive health evaluations. There is, instead, an overfocus on the disability so that the rest of the woman is ignored. Some health care facilities and providers are not prepared to assess or treat women with disabilities" (p. 433). It is hoped that the annual health visit described in Section 4103 (Medicare Coverage of Annual Wellness Visit Providing a Personalized Prevention Plan) will improve care for women with disabilities by attending to all aspects of prevention. Section 4104 (Removal of Barriers to Preventive Services in Medicare) calls for elimination of deductibles for approved preventive services and colorectal screening should assist in making comprehensive health evaluation standard for women with disabilities.

## Empirically Supported Treatment: Application to Women with Disabilities?

Banks (2012) reviewed critiques of the empirical basis of health treatments. The American Psychological Association's (2005) *Policy Statement on Evidence-Based Practice in Psychology* indicates that evidence-based treatment incorporates the best research evidence; clinical expertise; patient's specific problems, strengths, personality, sociocultural context, and preferences; and clinical implications. As noted by Dorsey and Graham (2011),

> Section 4302 of the Affordable Care Act establishes a roadmap for improving data collection efforts for racial and ethnic minorities, individuals with disabilities, and populations with limited English-language proficiency. The goal of the section is to improve efforts to reduce disparities through the standardization, collection, analysis, and reporting of data on health and health care disparities (p. 2379).

The ACA appears to maximize the definition of empirical support in Section 933 (Health Care Delivery System Research) to integrate research from multiple disciplines with information about treatment outcomes. However, in Section 511 (Maternal, Infant, and Early Childhood Home Visiting Programs), empirical support is described as "evaluated using well-designed and rigorous...randomized controlled research designs, and the evaluation results [that] have been published in a peer-reviewed journal; or...quasi-experimental research designs" (Patient Protection and Affordable

Care Act, 2010, pp. 571–572). Given the breadth of disabilities experienced by women, it will be important to ensure that research includes women with disabilities as participants and researchers, with attention to the necessity of culturally relevant adaptation of "empirically supported" treatment.

## USE OF TECHNOLOGY UNDER THE ACA

Routine health care for women is continuous throughout the life cycle; these needs are complex across many specialty areas. Moreover, women often bear the burden of caregiving for members of their family. The strong emphasis of the ACA on technology can prove beneficial to women as it creates challenges to transform our health care delivery system. If technology can be harnessed to facilitate integration and address complexity of needs, it can indeed be transformative. Already there are calls for software developers to create new apps for women's health. The U.S. Department of Health and Human Services (HHS) recently launched the Reducing Cancer Among Women of Color App Challenge. It calls on entrepreneurs to create an application for mobile devices that can help underserved and minority women fight and prevent cancer. The challenge is a first-of-its-kind effort to address health disparities among racial and ethnic minorities. HHS is particularly focused on reaching women who might not connect with traditional media sources, especially women of color, and their caregivers. Through the use of smartphone and computer apps, women and community health workers could have health care information at their fingertips to make informed health decisions. More than 300,000 new cases of breast, cervical, uterine, and ovarian cancer are diagnosed each year, according to the National Cancer Institute. Although the incidence and prevalence of these cancers are widespread, disparities in prevention, early treatment, quality of care, and outcomes result in a higher prevalence and mortality rates among minority and underserved women. "This app challenge is an example of our work to reduce health disparities, building on the HHS Action Plan to Reduce Racial and Ethnic Health Disparities," said J. Nadine Gracia, MD, MSCE, Acting Deputy Assistant Secretary for Minority Health. The app must be able to communicate with electronic health records used by their health care providers and other members of their health care teams, and protect patient privacy. Their vision is to:

1. Provide users with general, accessible information about preventive and screening services for breast and gynecologic cancers—in different languages and in culturally appropriate contexts.
2. Communicate with patient health records or provider-sponsored patient portals in a secure way that protects patient privacy and that will provide specific reminders and trigger electronic health record-based clinical decision support about preventive services.

3. Support the secure storage, viewing, and exchange of complex patient care plans in a way that protects patient privacy while strengthening communications between a patient's care team that might be located across a large geographic area, such as a local clinician being able to work with a regional cancer center in a major metropolitan area.
4. Support patient engagement and caregiver support by helping patients and their caregivers keep track of complex care plans with a particular emphasis on connections to community health workers.

The Reducing Cancer Among Women of Color App Challenge is a partnership between the Office of the National Coordinator for Health Information Technology and the HHS Office of Minority Health.

## WORKFORCE ISSUES

Although health care reform under the ACA makes progress in providing the framework for the integration of health and behavioral health care for women, the United States has not made significant progress in health care practice or reimbursement mechanisms; this must be supported by the following initiatives:

1. The health care team must include a behavioral health professional with referral and reimbursement mechanisms that support that model. The scope of behavioral health care goes beyond mental health and substance use disorders. Behavioral health care has many important implications for health interventions and treatment adherence, including such conditions as cancer or heart disease. Reimbursement mechanisms should allow fee for services from licensed behavioral health care specialists and doctoral-level mental health professionals independent of MDs; for instance, nurse practitioners or physician's assistants can provide services independent of MDs. For example, the Paul Wellstone and Pete Domenici Mental Health and Addiction Equity Act (2008) has ACA provisions in providing access to mental health services at parity in health insurance markets by January 1, 2014.
2. The current behavioral health workforce is insufficient in numbers and scope to support traditional mental health services for women and underserved minorities; it must be expanded to support the ACA. More behavioral education and training programs must be funded at the graduate and postdoctoral level. Funding for women and minority behavioral health care could include broadening the focus of the Minority Fellowship Program to include patient-focused health and mental health programs. The training of traditional health professions must also incorporate behavioral health care professionals as an essential part of the multidisciplinary

team, and in education and training, internships, and postdoctoral opportunities.

3. Provide line item funding and more funding support for behavioral health care translational research programs at all the National Institutes of Health institutes at the doctoral and postdoctoral levels.

## CONCLUSIONS

Health care reform under the ACA has significant implications for women's health. It can be transformative in integrating care delivery, currently fragmented between different systems of health and mental health care, between specialty care for different parts of a woman's body and life cycle health concerns, and between providers for different members of a woman's family. The focus of the ACA and its implementation should be on women patient-centered health care outcomes. Both legislative statutes and structural models such as the medical home model might help to achieve these outcomes.

## REFERENCES

AFP-Relaxnews. (2012, September 21). Some women lack knowledge about contraceptives. *New York Daily News*. Retrieved from www.nydailynews.com

American Psychological Association. (2005). *Policy statement on evidence-based practice in psychology*. Retrieved from http://www.apa.org/practice/resources/evidence/evidence-based-statement.pdf

American Psychological Association. (2007). *Report of the APA task force on socio-economic status*. Washington, DC: Author.

Americans with Disabilities Act of 1990, as Amended 2008, 42 U.S.C.A. 12101 *et seq.*

Banks, M. E. (2007). Women with disabilities, Domestic violence against. In N. A. Jackson (Ed.), *Encyclopedia of domestic violence*, (pp. 723–728). New York, NY: Taylor & Francis.

Banks, M. E. (2010). 2009 Division 35 presidential address: Feminist psychology and women with disabilities: An emerging alliance. *Psychology of Women Quarterly*, *34*, 431–442. doi:10.1111/j.1471-6402.2010.01593.x

Banks, M. E. (2012). Multiple minority identities and mental health: Social and research implications of diversity within and between groups. In R. Nettles & R. Balter (Eds.), *Multiple minority identities: Applications for practice, research, and training*, (pp. 35–58). New York, NY: Springer.

Banks, M. E. (2013). The therapeutic needs of culturally diverse individuals with physical disabilities. In F. A. Paniagua & A.-M. Yamada (Eds.), *Handbook of multicultural mental health*, (2nd ed., pp. 463–482). Amsterdam, The Netherlands: Elsevier.

Banks, M. E., & Marshall, C. (2004). Beyond the "triple-whammy": Social class as a factor in discrimination against persons with disabilities. In J. L. Chin (Ed.), *The psychology of prejudice and discrimination: Combating prejudice and all forms of discrimination. Vol. 4: Disability, religion, physique, and other traits*, (pp. 95–110). Westport, CT: Praeger.

Borneman, T. (2009). Foreword. In C. A. Marshall, E. Kendall, M. E. Banks, & R. M. S. Gover (Eds.), *Disabilities: Insights from across fields and around the world: Vol. 1: The experience: Definitions, causes, and consequences*, (pp. ix–xi). Westport, CT: Praeger.

Braun, K., Yee, B. W. K., Brown, C. V., & Mokuau, N. (2004). Native Hawaiian and Pacific Islander elders. In K. E. Whitfield (Ed.), *Closing the gap: Improving the health of minority elders in the new millennium*, (pp. 55–67). Washington, DC: Minority Taskforce, Gerontological Society of America.

Chan, V. H.-C. (2012, December 2). Female fights: #1 Sandra Fluke. *Yahoo! News.* Retrieved from http://news.yahoo.com/year-in-review-2012-female-fights-sandra-fluke-003412756.html

Croghan, T. W., & Brown, J. D. (2010). *Integrating mental health treatment into the patient centered medical home* (AHRQ Publication No. 10-0084-EF). Washington, DC: Agency for Healthcare Research and Quality, U.S. Department of Health and Human Services.

Dong, X. Q., Chang, E. S., Wong, E., & Simon, M. (2012). The perceptions, social determinants, and negative health outcomes associated with depressive symptoms among U.S. Chinese older adults. *The Gerontologist, 52*, 650–663.

Dorsey, R., & Graham, G. (2011). New HHS data standards for race, ethnicity, sex, primary language, and disability status. *JAMA: Journal of the American Medical Association, 306*, 2378–2379. doi:10.1001/jama.2011.1789

Families USA. (2012). *Being a woman just got a little easier: How the Affordable Care Act benefits women*. Retrieved from http://www.familiesusa.org/resources/publications/fact-sheets/being-a-woman-just-got-a.html

Feinberg, L., Reinhard, S. C., Houser, A., & Chula, R. (2011). *Valuing the invaluable: 2011 update. The growing contributions and costs of family caregiving*. Retrieved from http://assets.aarp.org/rgcenter/ppi/ltc/i51-caregiving.pdf

Goodwin, M. (2012, August 21). Legitimate rape—A dangerous fallacy. *The Chronicle of Higher Education*. Retrieved from http://chronicle.com/blogs/conversation/2012/08/21/legitimate-rape-a-dangerous-fallacy/

Goudreau, J. (2010). *What the health care bill means for women*. Retrieved from http://www.forbes.com/2010/03/23/health-care-bill-peolosi-forbes-woman-well-being-health-insurance-expenses.html

Jarrett, E. M., Yee, B. W. K., & Banks, M. E. (2007). Benefits of comprehensive health care for improving health outcomes in women. *Professional Psychology: Research and Practice, 38*, 305–313. doi:10.1037/0735-7028.38.3.305

Kaye, H. S. (2003). *Improved employment opportunities for people with disabilities* (Disability Statistics Report No. 17). Washington, DC: U.S. Department of Education, National Institute on Disability and Rehabilitation Research.

Kim, H., Chang, M., Rose, K., & Kim, S. (2011). Predictors of caregiver burden in caregivers of individuals with dementia. *Journal of Advanced Nursing, 68*, 846–855.

Korb, L., & Arons, J. (2012). Women in military deserve better care. *Politico.* Retrieved from http://www.politico.com/news/stories/0912/81604.html

MetLife Mature Market Institute. (2011, June). *The MetLife study of caregiving costs to working caregivers: Double jeopardy for baby boomers caring for their parents.*

Retrieved from https://www.metlife.com/assets/cao/mmi/publications/studies/2011/mmi-caregiving-costs-working-caregivers.pdf

Moore, L. (2012, August 20). Rep. Todd Akin: The statement and the reaction. *New York Times*. Retrieved from http://www.nytimes.com/2012/08/21/us/politics/rep-todd-akin-legitimate-rape-statement-and-reaction.html?_r=0

National Alliance for Caregiving in collaboration with AARP. (2009). *Caregiving in the U.S.: A focused look at the ethnicity of those caring for someone age 50 or older. Executive summary*. Retrieved from http://www.caregiving.org/pdf/research/FINAL_EthnicExSum_formatted_w_toc.pdf

National Alliance for Caregiving. (2011, November). *Caregiving costs. Declining health in the Alzheimer's caregiver as dementia increases in the care recipient*. Retrieved from http://www.caregiving.org/pdf/research/Alzheimers_Caregiving_Costs_Study_FINAL.pdf

Newcomer, R. J., Kang, T., & Doty, P. (2011). Allowing spouses to be paid personal care providers: Spouse availability and effects on Medicaid-funded service use and expenditures. *The Gerontologist, 52*, 517–530.

Nosek, M. A., Foley, C. C., Hughes, R. B., & Howland, C. A. (2001). Vulnerabilities for abuse among women with disabilities. *Sexuality and Disability, 19*, 177–189.

Patient Protection and Affordable Care Act, Pub. L. No. 111–148 (2010).

Paul Wellstone and Pete Domenici Mental Health and Addiction Equity Act. (2008). Retrieved from http://www.cms.gov/Regulations-and-Guidance/Health-Insurance-Reform/HealthInsReformforConsume/downloads/MHPAEA.pdf

Sanchez, K., Chapa, T., Ybarra, R., & Martinez, O. N. (2012). *Eliminating disparities through the integration of behavioral health and primary care services for racial and ethnic minorities, including populations with limited English proficiency: A review of the literature*. Washington, DC: U.S. Department of Health and Human Services, Office of Minority Health & the Hogg Foundation for Mental Health.

Shen, A. (2012). 2012 Republican platform to advocate abortion ban without rape exception. *Think Progress*. Retrieved from http://thinkprogress.org/election/2012/08/21/718461/2012-republican-platform-to-advocate-abortion-ban-without-rape-exception/?mobile=nc

Yancura, L. A. (2013). Justifications for caregiving in White, Asian American, and Native Hawaiian grandparents raising grandchildren. *Journals of Gerontology: Series B: Psychological Sciences and Social Sciences, 68*, 139–144. doi:10.1093/geronb/gbs098

Yee, B. W. K., DeBaryshe, B., Yuen, S., Kim, S. Y., & McCubbin, H. (2006). Asian American and Pacific Islander families: Resiliency and life-span socialization in a cultural context. In F. T. L. Leong, A. G. Inman, A. Ebreo, L. H. Yang, & L. M. F. Kinoshita (Eds.), *Handbook of Asian American psychology*, (2nd ed., pp. 69–86). Thousand Oaks, CA: Sage.

# The Impact of the Affordable Care Act on Behavioral Health Care for Individuals From Racial and Ethnic Communities

OSCAR MORGAN, FORD KURAMOTO, WILLIAM EMMET,
JUDY L. STANGE, and ERIC NOBUNAGA

*Magna Systems, Inc., Los Angeles, California, USA*

*The lack of health care insurance disproportionally affects individuals from racial and ethnic minority communities with chronic, yet in some instances, preventable health conditions. The Affordable Care Act (ACA) will provide insurance coverage to an additional 32 million Americans not currently insured. More than half of these additional insured include racial and ethnic minorities. The ACA not only reduces financial barriers to health care, but also improves access to quality behavioral health care for all. This article describes the benefits and impact of the ACA on individuals from racial and ethnic communities.*

The Patient Protection and Affordable Care Act, commonly called the Affordable Care Act (ACA), expands access to health care, improves the quality of care, and has the potential to reduce health disparities that affect racial and ethnic minority communities. The ACA addresses health disparities through holistic approaches that take into account all aspects of an individual's needs, including psychological, physical, and social, to improve the overall quality of life. The broad policy agenda envisioned by the ACA addresses many of the issues delineated in the Institute of Medicine (IOM) report, *Unequal Treatment: Confronting Racial and Ethnic Disparities in Health Care* (Smedley, Stith, & Nelson, 2003). The report synthesized a large body of research that demonstrated the severity of health disparities affecting racial and ethnic minorities.

To address the disparities reported by the IOM report, the ACA calls for the expansion of health care insurance and public health programs, an increase in preventive health care, health promotion, the integration of primary and behavioral health care, culturally competent and linguistically appropriate services, and an increase in the number and diversity of the health care workforce. Furthermore, the ACA seeks to address health care disparities through better data collection, a focus on cultural and linguistic competence of providers, and increased research on the development of evidence-based practices.

People of color from racial and ethnic minority populations have disproportionately more preventable health conditions than the general population and are more likely to be uninsured, due to poverty status and other social determinants of health. The ACA health insurance coverage will help eliminate barriers to gaining access to health care through Medicaid expansion and the health insurance exchanges. The ACA has the potential for providing high-quality, affordable health and behavioral health services that can improve health status, promote improved quality of life, and reduce health disparities for people of color.

The ACA and health care reform alone cannot address all the factors that contribute to racial and ethnic health disparities. However, the ACA applies an integrative and collaborative approach that will help identify the social determinants of health that impact the health and well-being of ethnic and racial communities. These social determinants might include low socioeconomic status, lack of educational opportunities, inadequate housing, and exposure to violence and crime.

As the U.S. population continues to shift toward greater racial and ethnic diversity, the ACA provides an opportunity for the health care system to respond to the growing body of evidence indicating that culture, language, and lifestyle affect health conditions. Language has been described as medicine's most essential technology, the principle instrument for conducting its work (Bowen & Canada, 2001). Language barriers between the providers and consumers that result in abbreviated or erroneous communication can lead to poor and ineffective decision making. Consequently it becomes imperative that health care providers strive for linguistic competence when communicating with our increasingly diverse populations. Clearly understood communications enables all parties to determine the most effective approach to prevention, diagnosis, and treatment.

## THE CHANGING FACE OF THE UNITED STATES AND IMPLICATIONS OF ACA HEALTH CARE COVERAGE

Over the last decade, the racial and ethnic makeup of the United States has undergone a dramatic change. The 2010 census counted 196.8 million

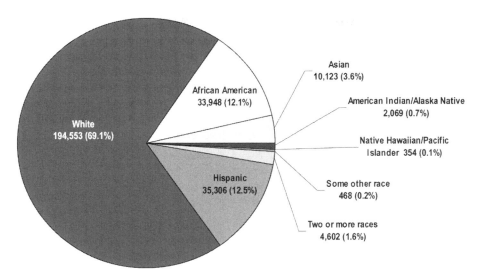

**FIGURE 1** U.S. population, by race and ethnicity, 2000 (×1,000). *Source:* Pew Research Center (2011). (Color figure available online.)

individuals in the White population, or 63.7% of the total U.S. population (see Figures 1 and 2). The Hispanic population grew by 43%, from a total of 35.3 million in the 2000 census to 50.5 million in 2010. This growth makes Hispanics the nation's largest minority group, at 16.3% of the total population. Among other ethnic minority groups, the 2010 census also counted 37.7 million African Americans (12.2%), 14.5 million Asians

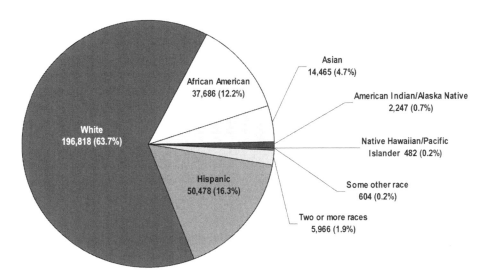

**FIGURE 2** U.S. population, by race and ethnicity, 2010 (×1,000). *Source:* Pew Research Center (2011). (Color figure available online.)

(4.7%), 2.2 million American Indians and Alaskan Natives (about 1%), and 482,000 Native Hawaiians and Pacific Islanders (less than 1%). Six million non-Hispanic Whites, or 1.9% of the U.S. population, identified themselves in the census as more than one race (Pew Research Center, 2011). At this growth rate, the children of racial and ethnic minority populations will account for over half of all persons under 18 years by 2019 (Kurtz, 2013).

The U.S. Census data from 2000 to 2010 indicates that the non-Hispanic White population made up only 8.3% of the total growth, whereas racial and ethnic minorities accounted for an overwhelming 91.7% of the nation's population growth. Hispanics made up 56% of this 91.7% of growth, and other racial and ethnic minorities made up 35.7% of the growth (see Figure 3). Furthermore, the U.S. Census Bureau projects that by 2050, racial and ethnic minorities will become the majority population at 54% (CNN, 2008).

Populations vary by race and ethnicities in their distribution across states. Table 1 lists the largest populations of racial and ethnic groups and the White population by selected states. Not surprisingly, the largest numbers in each of the ethnic minority groups, except African Americans, live in California. For example, 33% of all Asian Americans and 28% of all Hispanic/Latinos living in the United States reside in California. One of the challenges in aggregating racial and ethnic demographic and other data is the

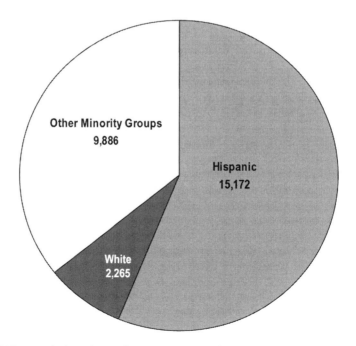

**FIGURE 3** U.S. population change between 2000 and 2010, by race and ethnicity (×1,000). *Source:* Pew Research Center (2011). (Color figure available online.)

**TABLE 1** Top 10 States with Largest Estimated Resident Population by Race and Hispanic Origin (Population × 1,000)

| Rank | African American | | | American Indian/ Alaska Native | | | Asian American | | | Hispanic/Latino[a] | | | Native Hawaiian and Pacific Islander | | | White | | |
|---|---|---|---|---|---|---|---|---|---|---|---|---|---|---|---|---|---|---|
| Total | | 40,751 | | | 3,815 | | | 15,578 | | | 52,045 | | | 692 | | | 243,470 | |
| 1 | NY | 3,401 | 8.3% | CA | 637 | 16.7% | CA | 5,142 | 33.0% | CA | 14,360 | 27.6% | CA | 185 | 26.8% | CA | 27,883 | 11.5% |
| 2 | FL | 3,142 | 7.7% | AZ | 340 | 8.9% | NY | 1,518 | 9.7% | TX | 9,792 | 18.8% | HI | 138 | 20.0% | TX | 20,769 | 8.5% |
| 3 | TX | 3,139 | 7.7% | OK | 338 | 8.9% | TX | 1,039 | 6.7% | FL | 4,356 | 8.4% | WA | 44 | 6.4% | FL | 14,959 | 6.1% |
| 4 | GA | 3,045 | 7.5% | TX | 263 | 6.9% | NJ | 766 | 4.9% | NY | 3,495 | 6.7% | TX | 33 | 4.8% | NY | 13,910 | 5.7% |
| 5 | CA | 2,505 | 6.1% | NM | 210 | 5.5% | IL | 619 | 4.0% | IL | 2,080 | 4.0% | UT | 27 | 3.9% | PA | 10,673 | 4.4% |
| 6 | NC | 2,121 | 5.2% | NY | 185 | 4.9% | HI | 530 | 3.4% | AZ | 1,949 | 3.7% | NY | 25 | 3.6% | IL | 10,042 | 4.1% |
| 7 | IL | 1,906 | 4.7% | NC | 149 | 3.9% | WA | 509 | 3.3% | NJ | 1,601 | 3.1% | FL | 20 | 2.9% | OH | 9,654 | 4.0% |
| 8 | MD | 1,749 | 4.3% | WA | 125 | 3.3% | FL | 494 | 3.2% | CO | 1,071 | 2.1% | NV | 20 | 2.8% | MI | 7,925 | 3.3% |
| 9 | VA | 1,600 | 3.9% | AK | 107 | 2.8% | VA | 466 | 3.0% | NM | 973 | 1.9% | AZ | 17 | 2.4% | NC | 6,966 | 2.9% |
| 10 | LA | 1,482 | 3.6% | FL | 93 | 2.4% | MA | 371 | 2.4% | GA | 892 | 1.7% | OR | 15 | 2.2% | NJ | 6,540 | 2.7% |

*Note. Source:* Table 4. Estimates of the Resident Population by Race and Hispanic Origin for the United States and States: July 1, 2011 (SC-EST2011-04), U.S. Census Bureau, Population Division, May 2012.

[a]According to the U.S. Census, Hispanic origin is considered an ethnicity, not a race. Hispanics may be of any race.

complexity of finding and interpreting information for the four major groups. For example, according to the U.S. Census, Hispanic origin is considered an ethnicity and not a race. Other Census categories, such as Asian Americans, are very diverse and made up of more than 30 different subgroups. The way Asian American data are presented can be misleading because they are often not disaggregated. When the data are not disaggregated, they mask the differences among the subgroups, such as the high rate of poverty among Southeast Asians.

Figure 4 shows the estimated populations of the former U.S. territories: the six Pacific Island Jurisdictions, Puerto Rico, and the U.S. Virgin Islands. Although small in numbers compared to most states in the Continental United States, this information was included because the indigenous populations of the territories are primarily people of color, such as the Hispanic population in Puerto Rico. Some of these territories will participate in the ACA. As with members of these racial and ethnic minority populations living in the Continental United States, those living in the eight territories have severe health and behavioral health care needs. As a result, the potential benefits of the ACA are important to them. At this point, Puerto Rico is the only territory intending to create its own health insurance exchange (Pernas, 2012).

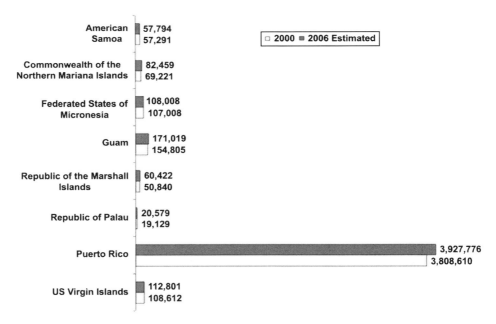

**FIGURE 4** Population of the Pacific Island jurisdictions, Puerto Rico, and U.S. Virgin Islands. *Source:* Pacificweb.org (see http://pacificweb.org/categories/Statistical%20Activities/Statistical Activities.html), U.S. Census Bureau (2006), and U.S. Virgin Islands Bureau of Economic Research (2009). (Color figure available online.)

The Virgin Islands, Guam, American Samoa, and the Commonwealth of the Northern Mariana Islands have not applied for a health insurance exchange at this time. They might be able to receive an additional Medicaid allocation if they do not have an exchange (DeJongh, 2010).

Figure 4 shows the wide variations in population size among the territories. For example, Puerto Rico has the largest population at almost 4 million compared to the Republic of Palau with the smallest population of about 21,000. Each entity has its own unique history, language, culture, and political and economic issues. They also have differing formal relationships with the United States, some through compacts of free association (Pacific Island Health Officers' Association, 2013). Three entities are sovereign nations: the Federated States of Micronesia, the Republic of the Marshall Islands, and the Republic of Palau. The territories are made up of hundreds of islands and atolls widely distributed geographically around the globe in the Caribbean, South Pacific, and across Micronesia to the area near the Philippines.

To fully address racial and ethnic minority issues vis-à-vis the ACA, we must also recognize the significance of institutionalized populations, particularly those incarcerated in jails and prisons. The statistics provided by the U.S. Census Bureau understate the size and needs of some racial and ethnic populations in the United States due to the way the U.S. Census Bureau collects population data. The U.S. Census Bureau normally collects data for households and does not always include homeless individuals or institutionalized individuals, such as those in jails and prisons. However, in the past 15 years, jail and prison populations have increased dramatically. A recent estimate of the total incarcerated population indicates that each year as many as 10 million persons move through the U.S. correctional systems (Phillips, 2012). The United States has the highest incarceration rate in the world (Glaze, 2011). Of these incarcerated individuals, approximately 60% are racial and ethnic minorities, although they represent only 30% of the total U.S. population. Men in these populations are incarcerated at disproportionately higher rates: 1 in every 15 African American men and 1 in every 36 Hispanic men compared to 1 in every 106 White men (Kerby, 2012).

Due to the disproportionate numbers of incarcerated men of color, comprehensive data on incarcerated individuals would help us to better understand the impact of those numbers on racial and ethnic minority populations. Additionally, more comprehensive data would better reflect the positive impact the ACA might have on providing health and behavioral health services to incarcerated individuals, as well as follow-up on reentry in the community. Incarcerated individuals are more likely to have behavioral health problems (e.g., mental health and substance use disorders), communicable diseases (e.g., hepatitis C and HIV infection), and chronic illness health problems (e.g., diabetes and hypertension). About 50% of all the people in jails and prisons have mental health problems and 65% have alcohol or other drug abuse and addiction, conditions that are associated with recidivism.

Repeated incarcerations and the large numbers of individuals involved result in higher operating costs for the jails and prisons. Adequate health and behavioral health care services for these populations can reduce recidivism, as well as the high costs of health-related care in the criminal justice system (Phillips, 2012).

Local and state governments will continue to bear the costs of health care in jails and prisons. However, on release into the community, the ACA makes additional health and behavioral health care services available to the inmates. Keeping these individuals enrolled in ACA is a critical step to reducing recidivism and stopping the revolving door through the prison system. Pretrial detainees eligible for ACA enrollment and those already enrolled will remain insured until sentenced to incarceration. Medicaid eligibility, whether the result of ACA Medicaid expansion or enrollment in "traditional" Medicaid, can be suspended rather than terminated while an individual is in jail or prison to avoid the lengthy reapplication process on release. Eligible individuals could also apply for Medicaid while incarcerated to access needed services on reentry into the community (Phillips, 2012). Increased access to health and behavioral health services through the ACA, particularly for racial and ethnic minority populations, will improve prevention, improve treatment outcomes, and reduce recidivism and overall costs.

Racial and ethnic minorities suffer disproportionately from the negative impact of many health issues. The tables that follow provide context to the discussion on the implications of the ACA for improved health, behavioral health, and well-being among racial and ethnic minorities. They present an overview of selected demographic data, characteristics, and health issues that disproportionately and negatively affect these populations. Table 2 presents demographic data on educational attainment, language fluency, economic conditions, and health insurance coverage. Table 3 lists various health conditions and health disparities. Table 4 focuses on mental health conditions and related issues. Table 5 addresses substance use disorders, including the use of alcohol, tobacco and illicit drugs.

Table 2 illustrates the diversity among these population groups and points out that due to the nature of the collected data, comparable data are not always available for all groups. One common factor with both Hispanic/Latino and Asian American populations is the high percentages of bilingual persons, an important factor in language access and the delivery of culturally competent, high-quality services. The racial and ethnic minority populations also have relatively high rates of uninsured persons, discussed in a later section. The educational attainment data indicate that most of these populations have relatively low levels of attainment for high school and college graduation. Educational attainment is important because of its potential for higher personal incomes and socioeconomic class in the long term.

Language fluency also affects educational attainment, employment opportunities, and access to health and behavioral health services. Table 2

## THE AFFORDABLE CARE ACT AND INTEGRATED BEHAVIORAL HEALTH CARE

**TABLE 2** Demographic Profile

| Topic | African American | American Indian/ Alaska Native | Asian American | Hispanic/ Latino[a] | Native Hawaiian and Pacific Islander |
|---|---|---|---|---|---|
| Population, 2011 | | | | | |
| Total | 43.9 million, 14% | 6.3 million, 2% | 18.2 million, 6% | 52 million, 17% | 1.4 million, 0.4% |
| Educational attainment | | | | | |
| High school graduate | 82% | 77% | 85% | 62% | 89% |
| College graduate | 16% male, 20% female | 13% | 50% | 13% | 20% |
| Language fluency | | | | | |
| Speak another language at home | ❶ | 28% | 77% | 76% | 30% |
| Nonfluent in English | ❶ | ❷ | 36% | 35% | ❷ |
| Economics | | | | | |
| Family median income | $39,988 | $39,664 | $76,736 | $40,165 | $56,521 |
| Poverty level | 27% | 28% | 13% | 25% | 17% |
| Unemployment, 2011 | 15.9% | 14.6% | 7.0% | 11.5% | 10.4% |

*Note.* ❶ = English is predominant language; ❷ = Data not available or not collected.
[a]Hispanic origin is considered by the U.S. Census as an ethnicity, not a race. Hispanics may be of any race.

illustrates that Asian Americans and Hispanic/Latino populations have similar rates of speaking a language other than English at home (77% and 76%, respectively) and not being fluent in English (36% and 35%, respectively). American Indian/Alaskan Natives and Native Hawaiians and Pacific Islanders also have significant rates of speaking another language at home (28% and 30%, respectively).

Living in poverty is a social determinant that negatively affects health and behavioral health status. Table 2 shows that most of the racial and ethnic groups have high rates of poverty. Note that because the Asian American data are not disaggregated, they mask the high rates of poverty among certain subgroups, such as Hmong. The poverty rate among American Indians/ Alaskan Natives is 28%, African Americans 27% and Hispanic/Latinos 25%. The ACA might not, by itself, lift these people out of poverty, but providing effective health and behavioral health care will help a great deal to promote healthier, more productive, and longer life spans for these groups.

Table 3 lists the 10 leading causes of death, special health issues and risk factors, and health disparities. It shows relatively high rates of certain causes of death, such as unintentional injuries among American Indians/Alaskan Natives and Hispanics/Latinos and homicides among African Americans.

**TABLE 3** Health Conditions

| Topic | African American | American Indian/ Alaska Native | Asian American | Hispanic/Latino[a] | Native Hawaiian and Pacific Islander |
|---|---|---|---|---|---|
| 10 leading causes of death | Heart disease<br>Cancer<br>Stroke<br>Diabetes<br>Unintentional injuries<br>Kidney disease<br>Respiratory disease<br>Homicide<br>Septicemia<br>Alzheimer's | Heart disease<br>Cancer<br>Unintentional injuries<br>Diabetes<br>Liver disease and cirrhosis<br>Respiratory diseases<br>Stroke<br>Influenza, pneumonia<br>Kidney disease | Cancer<br>Heart disease<br>Stroke<br>Unintentional injuries<br>Diabetes<br>Influenza, pneumonia<br>Respiratory diseases<br>Kidney disease<br>Alzheimer's<br>Suicide | Cancer<br>Heart disease<br>Unintentional injuries<br>Stroke<br>Diabetes<br>Liver disease and cirrhosis<br>Respiratory diseases<br>Influenza, pneumonia<br>Homicide<br>Kidney disease | Cancer<br>Heart disease<br>Stroke<br>Unintentional injuries<br>Diabetes<br>Influenza, pneumonia<br>Respiratory diseases<br>Kidney disease<br>Alzheimer's<br>Suicide |
| Special health issues, risks | Maternal and infant health<br>Teen pregnancy<br>Asthma<br>High blood pressure<br>Smoking<br>Obesity<br>High cholesterol<br>Nutrition<br>Physical activity<br>Influenza<br>HIV/AIDS | Teen pregnancy<br>Infant mortality<br>HIV/AIDS<br>Obesity<br>Diabetes<br>Mental health<br>Alcohol<br>Smoking | HIV/AIDS<br>Hepatitis B<br>Smoking<br>Tuberculosis<br>Risk of gestational diabetes for mothers is higher than other groups<br>Rate of pregnancy related deaths is higher than Whites | Asthma<br>Chagas disease<br>HIV/AIDS<br>Teen pregnancy<br>Smoking<br>Infant mortality | Alcohol<br>Hepatitis B<br>HIV/AIDS<br>Obesity<br>Smoking<br>Tuberculosis<br>High rates of infant mortality in the Pacific Islands |

| Health disparities | | | | | |
| --- | --- | --- | --- | --- | --- |
| Women/men ages 45–74 had highest death rates from heart disease and stroke<br>Infant mortality rate twice as high as infants of Whites<br>Highest death rate from homicide for ages 15–59<br>HIV rate was the highest of all groups | Mothers had second highest infant mortality rate<br>Highest rate of motor-vehicle-related deaths, one of the highest rates of suicides, and the second highest death rate due to drug abuse<br>Among the highest prevalence of binge drinking<br>Youth 12–17 years and adults aged 18 years or older had the highest prevalence of current smoking | In 2010, were least likely to have had a Pap test (68.0%)<br>In 2008, hepatitis B incidence was 1.6 times greater than Whites<br>High rates of tuberculosis<br>High risk of gestational diabetes<br>High rates of pregnancy-related deaths | More likely to reside in counties that did not meet health standard for ozone<br>Lower influenza vaccination coverage among all persons aged >6 months<br>Males aged ≤20 years, obesity was highest among Mexican Americans<br>High rate of HIV diagnoses<br>Low birthweight babies 60% higher for Puerto Ricans than Whites<br>Puerto Ricans have high rates of asthma, HIV/AIDS, infant mortality<br>Mexican Americans have high rates of diabetes | High cancer death rates<br>Relative survival rate for all cancers is 47%, compared with 57% for Whites and 55% for all races<br>Infant mortality rate was 9.6 per 1,000 live births<br>Prevalence of diabetes was 3 times greater than Whites<br>Incidence of hepatitis B was 1.6 times greater than Whites<br>High rates of smoking, alcohol consumption, and obesity<br>High incidence of HIV infection<br>High percentage of populations residing in counties with air quality that does not meet EPA standards |

[a]Hispanic origin is considered by the U.S. Census as an ethnicity, not a race. Hispanics may be of any race.

**TABLE 4** Mental Health Conditions

| Topic | African American | American Indian/ Alaska Native | Asian American | Hispanic/ Latino[a] | Native Hawaiian and Pacific Islander |
|---|---|---|---|---|---|
| Serious psychological distress | High psychological distress due to poverty 20% more likely than Whites | | 70% of Southeast Asians diagnosed with posttraumatic stress disorder | High psychological distress due to poverty | |
| Suicide rate | Rate of 5.2 (per 100,000); men is four times higher than for women | Rate of 17.5 (per 100,000) Second leading cause of death for ages 10–34 | Rate of 6.1 (per 100,000) 10th leading cause of death Older Asian American women have the highest suicide rate of all women over 65 years in United States | Rate of 5.9 (per 100,000) Rate for men is five times higher than women and four times higher for adolescent females compared to Whites | A leading cause of death: Pacific Islander youth living in the islands have high rates of suicide |
| Violent deaths | Homicide is the leading cause of death among 10–24-year-olds Highest homicide rates for males between 20–24 years Homicide rate of 18.8 per 100,000 (age adjusted) in 2009 | 75% of all deaths between age 11–21, including unintentional injuries, homicide, and suicide Homicide is the third leading cause of death Homicide rate of 7.1 per 100,000 (age adjusted) in 2009 | Homicide rate was 2.2 per 100,000 (age adjusted) in 2009 | Homicide is the second leading cause of death among 10–24-year-olds Homicide rate was 6.2 per 100,000 (age adjusted) in 2009 | Homicide rate was 2.2 per 100,000 (age adjusted) in 2009 |

[a]Hispanic origin is considered by the U.S. Census as an ethnicity, not a race. Hispanics may be of any race.

In terms of special health issues and risk factors, alcohol use was high on the list for Native Hawaiians and Pacific Islanders, hepatitis B for Asian Americans, and Chagas disease (an infection spread by insects) for Hispanics/Latinos. Health disparities and the rates for them among the racial and ethnic groups varied widely, including the highest homicide death rate for African Americans, second highest infant mortality rate for American Indians/Alaskan Natives, high rates of tuberculosis among Asian Americans, high rates of HIV diagnosis among Hispanics/Latinos, and high rates of diabetes among Native Hawaiians and Pacific Islanders.

Table 4 shows the mental health conditions affecting the ethnic minority groups under discussion. The available data provided in Table 4 illustrate a high level of psychological distress for some of the racial and ethnic groups. These groups have high rates of suicide and violent deaths (e.g., homicides among African Americans and Hispanics/Latinos).

Table 5 illustrates comparative rates of substance use disorders among the groups, showing that substance use disorders affect all of the groups. Underage alcohol use was 23% among Hispanics/Latinos, 20% for American Indians/Alaskan Natives, 19% for Asian Americans, and 18% for African Americans. Binge drinking was highest among Hispanics/Latinos at 23% and tobacco use (among those 12 years and older) was highest among American Indians/Alaskan Natives at 43%.

Tables 2 through 5 identify demographic, health, and behavioral health characteristics of the racial and ethnic minority groups in the Continental United States and the territories. These characteristics indicate the need for improved health and behavioral health care for racial and ethnic minorities.

**TABLE 5** Substance Use Disorders

| Topic | African American | American Indian/Alaska Native | Asian American | Hispanic/Latino[a] | Native Hawaiian and Pacific Islander |
|---|---|---|---|---|---|
| Past month use, illicit drugs, 12 or older | 10.0% | 13.4% | 3.8% | 8.4% | 11.0% |
| Alcohol use in past month, ages 12–20 | 18.1% | 20.0% | 18.8% | 22.5% | Not provided |
| Current binge alcohol use | 19.4% | 15.2% | 11.6% | 23.4% | Not provided |
| Current binge alcohol use, ages 12–20 | 9.4% | 13.9% | 9.1% | 14.0% | Not provided |
| Current tobacco use, 12 and older | 26.2% | 43.0% | 13.0% | 20.4% | Not provided |
| Substance dependence or abuse, 2011 | 7.2% | 16.8% | 3.3% | 8.7% | 10.6% |

[a]Hispanic origin is considered by the U.S. Census as an ethnicity, not a race. Hispanics may be of any race.

## MEDICAID EXPANSION

How will the ACA help meet these needs identified in Tables 2 through 5? One major way the ACA will meet these needs is by making available about $952 billion in Medicaid funds for the Medicaid expansion provisions (Holahan, Buettgens, Carroll, & Dorn, 2012). These funds will extend benefits to low-income citizens up to 138% of the federal poverty level. About 59% of the individuals that will be newly insured through the Medicaid expansion will be racial and ethnic minorities. However, at this time, 26 states (see Figure 5) will not implement the ACA Medicaid expansion provision because of actions taken by their governors and state legislators. The map in Figure 5 indicates current state plans for Medicaid expansion.

Table 6 lists the states that not only have the highest number of uninsured individuals, but also do not plan to implement the Medicaid expansion and other provisions of the ACA. The states in descending order of the percentage of total uninsured persons are shown in Table 6.

Table 7 lists the states with the highest overall rates of nonelderly uninsured by race and ethnicity. Note that the total rate of uninsured by race and ethnicity was highest among Hispanic populations (31%), followed by African Americans (19%), Asian/Pacific Islanders (17%), and Whites (13%). Certain groups within some of the states had even higher rates of uninsured, such as Hispanic populations in Georgia (45%), followed by Asian/Pacific Islanders in Louisiana (33%), African Americans in West Virginia (29%), and Whites in Florida (19%).

Table 8 provides an estimate of the rates of nonelderly uninsured by state and race and ethnic group with incomes up to 138% of the federal poverty level. Table 8 identifies the potential rates of persons who could become eligible for health insurance through the Medicaid expansion by selected states beginning in October 2013.

The group with the highest total rate is African Americans (64%), followed by Hispanics (58%), Asian/Pacific Islanders (51%), and Whites (49). The African American population had the highest rate by state in Michigan (73%), followed by Hispanics in Alabama (70%), Asian/Pacific Islanders in Hawaii (64%), and Whites in Kentucky (60%). The high rate of nonelderly African Americans who might be eligible for insurance through the Medicaid expansion emphasizes the dramatically high rates of African Americans living in or near poverty. Health insurance for these populations of color has the potential for vastly improving their access to quality care; improving their individual, family, and community health status; and reducing health disparities, enhancing health equity, and controlling costs. Unfortunately, millions of low-income people of color are likely to remain without improved health coverage, primarily because their state governments decided not to participate in the Medicaid expansion (Alonso-Zaldivar, 2013).

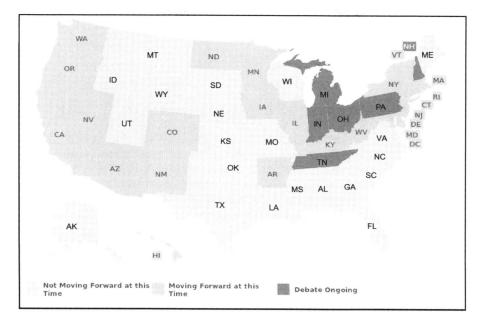

**FIGURE 5** Status of state action on Medicaid expansion (as of July 1, 2013). *Source:* Kaiser Family Foundation (2013). (Color figure available online.)

Figure 6 shows the estimated rates of uninsured persons currently receiving Medicaid and other public health services and the rates of persons currently with private health insurance through an employer or their own individual insurance by race. As Figure 6 shows, Hispanic, African American, and Native American/Alaskan Natives have the highest rates of uninsured persons and those receiving care through Medicaid and other public health services. This generally means they have the lowest incomes, highest unemployment, and the most jobs with little or no health insurance benefits.

The decision of some states to not implement the Medicaid expansion exacerbates the current inadequate access to health care for racial and ethnic

**TABLE 6** States with Highest Number of Uninsured

| State | Percent Uninsured |
| --- | --- |
| Texas | 28.8 |
| Louisiana | 24.0 |
| Florida | 22.8 |
| Georgia | 22.5 |
| Alaska | 21.8 |
| Mississippi | 21.7 |
| Oklahoma | 21.4 |

*Note. Source:* Gallup Poll, March 2013 (see http://www.gallup.com/poll/161153/texas-uninsured-rate-moves-further-away-states.aspx).

# THE AFFORDABLE CARE ACT AND INTEGRATED BEHAVIORAL HEALTH CARE

**TABLE 7** States with Highest Uninsured Rates Among Nonelderly by Race/Ethnicity, 2011

| Rank | White | | Black | | Hispanic | | Asian/Pacific Islander | |
|------|-------|-----|-------|-----|----------|-----|------------------------|-----|
| Total U.S. | 13% | | 19% | | 31% | | 17% | |
| 1 | Florida | 19% | West Virginia | 29% | Georgia | 45% | Louisiana | 33% |
| 2 | Montana | 19% | Florida | 26% | North Carolina | 44% | Arkansas | 32% |
| 3 | Arkansas | 18% | Oklahoma | 24% | Alabama | 44% | Alaska | 29% |
| 4 | Nevada | 18% | Louisiana | 23% | Tennessee | 43% | Georgia | 28% |
| 5 | West Virginia | 18% | Mississippi | 23% | Mississippi | 43% | South Carolina | 26% |
| 6 | Georgia | 17% | Nevada | 23% | South Carolina | 42% | Texas | 24% |
| 7 | Oklahoma | 17% | Texas | 22% | Louisiana | 42% | Florida | 24% |
| 8 | Mississippi | 17% | Georgia | 22% | Utah | 41% | Nevada | 22% |
| 9 | Texas | 16% | South Carolina | 22% | Texas | 37% | Colorado | 21% |
| 10 | South Carolina | 16% | Kentucky | 22% | Oklahoma | 37% | North Carolina | 19% |

*Note. Source:* Kaiser Commission on Medicaid and the Uninsured (2013).

minority communities. As a result, these states might perpetuate health disparities, poorer health status, and a greater burden of disease for people of color.

## ADDRESSING HEALTH EQUITY AND HEALTH DISPARITIES

The discussion in the previous section addressed the impact of being uninsured and not having access to the Medicaid expansion provisions of

**TABLE 8** States with Highest Share of Nonelderly Uninsured <138% Federal Poverty Level by Race or Ethnicity, 2011

| Rank | White | | Black | | Hispanic | | Asian/Pacific Islander | |
|------|-------|-----|-------|-----|----------|-----|------------------------|-----|
| Total U.S. | 49% | | 64% | | 58% | | 51% | |
| 1 | Kentucky | 60% | Michigan | 73% | Alabama | 70% | Hawaii | 64% |
| 2 | Hawaii | 59% | Alabama | 73% | Kentucky | 69% | Oklahoma | 63% |
| 3 | Alabama | 58% | South | 72% | Arkansas | 69% | Oregon | 58% |
| 4 | Tennessee | 56% | Mississippi | 72% | Missouri | 68% | Ohio | 57% |
| 5 | Georgia | 56% | Arkansas | 71% | Iowa | 68% | Michigan | 56% |
| 6 | Michigan | 55% | Kentucky | 70% | Indiana | 65% | California | 55% |
| 7 | Arkansas | 53% | Ohio | 69% | North | 64% | Tennessee | 55% |
| 8 | Oklahoma | 53% | Missouri | 69% | Ohio | 64% | Pennsylvania | 54% |
| 9 | Missouri | 53% | Kansas | 68% | Idaho | 64% | Minnesota | 53% |
| 10 | Ohio | 53% | Tennessee | 67% | Georgia | 63% | Louisiana | 52% |

*Note. Source:* Kaiser Commission on Medicaid and the Uninsured (2013).

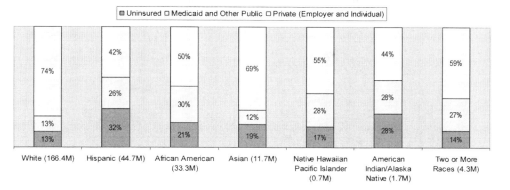

FIGURE 6 Health insurance coverage of nonelderly population by race/ethnicity, 2008. *Source:* Thomas and James (2009). (Color figure available online.)

the ACA on racial and ethnic minority communities. These factors have a negative impact on health equity and reducing health disparities, if the state policies remain unchanged. There are, however, additional factors that can contribute to health disparities. Undoubtedly access to appropriate health and behavioral health services is at the core of health equity and reducing health disparities. Even if individuals are financially insured by the ACA, they will need appropriate access to the care they need to reduce health disparities. Figures 7 and 8 illustrate the percentages of racial and ethnic minority groups and other populations that have no regular source of medical care or no doctor visits in the past year, respectively.

Figure 7 shows that most of the racial and ethnic minority populations have less regular access to medical care compared to the White populations, regardless of whether they are insured or uninsured. The same pattern exists in Figure 8 for no visits to a doctor in the past year.

Table 8 and Figures 6, 7, and 8 clearly demonstrate the existence of health disparities in terms of access to regular medical care and regular visits to a doctor. Basic access to regular medical care and regular visits to a doctor are, obviously, critical. Preventive care and early screening, diagnosis, and treatment cannot be provided without this access.

The ACA not only seeks to provide a means for individuals from racial and ethnic minority populations to pay for necessary prevention and treatment services, but also to improve the social, economic, and related conditions that affect the social determinants of health. For the ACA to have the greatest impact on social development and improving health outcomes across many domains, the services, programs, and policies must be based on the best science and culturally competent evidence.

To underscore the importance of using the most effective, evidence-based practices, the ACA provides $1.0 billion for comparative effectiveness research. One aspect of this research requires the development

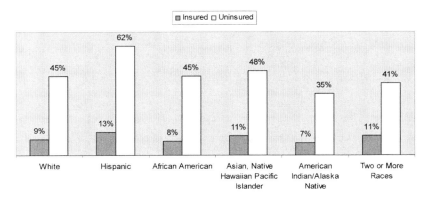

**FIGURE 7** Percent of nonelderly adults with no usual source of medical care, 2005–2006. *Source:* Thomas and James (2009). (Color figure available online.)

and expansion of methods to conduct timely, relevant research on evidence-based treatment for ethnic and racial communities. The ACA also requires the translation and dissemination of research findings, not only to practitioners, but also to diverse audiences of consumers and family members. The end goals are to increase the consumers' health care knowledge, provide timely information on evidence-based care, culturally appropriate treatments and practices, and help consumers or peers and practitioners make informed, relevant choices regarding their health care services and supports.

Although not common enough, there are evidenced-based as well as effective, culturally appropriate programs that provide models to emulate. Two examples of exemplary evidence-based programs that help develop effective youth prevention strategies as well as comprehensive, client-centered care for ethnic minority elderly include the Adverse Childhood Experience (ACE) Study and the Program of All-Inclusive Care for

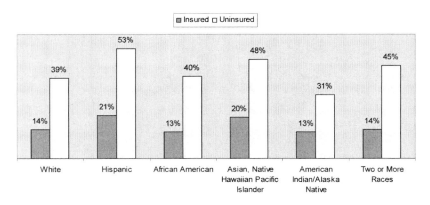

**FIGURE 8** Percentage of nonelderly adults with no doctor visit in past year, 2005–2006. *Source:* Thomas and James (2009). (Color figure available online.)

the Elderly (PACE). These programs demonstrate how fundamental aspects of the ACA, namely prevention, early intervention, service integration, and collaboration among health care professionals, can improve client outcomes.

The ACE Study is a joint effort between the Centers for Disease Control and Prevention (CDC) and Kaiser Permanente's Health Appraisal Clinic in San Diego. It shows that certain experiences involving social determinants of health are major risk factors for the leading causes of illness and death, as well as poor quality of life in the United States (CDC, 2103). The findings of this longitudinal study also suggest if such experiences or social determinants are addressed early, the onset of costly chronic diseases can be reduced, if not avoided entirely.

The On Lok model of care, pioneered in 1971 and now called PACE, allows ill or disabled Chinese seniors in the San Francisco Bay Area to continue living in their own homes and communities. PACE includes a core integrated multidisciplinary team of health professionals working in collaboration through a single point of access to provide individuals with preventive, primary, acute, rehabilitative, and long-term services. The integration and collaboration among the PACE culturally competent health care professionals results in the provision of culturally competent and linguistically appropriate, comprehensive care in a cost-effective manner (Hirth, Baskins, & Dever-Bumba, 2009).

## REDUCING HEALTH DISPARITIES BY ACA ENROLLMENT AND PARTICIPATION

It is anticipated that the number of individuals purchasing coverage through the health insurance marketplace will result in a significantly lower overall cost of insurance premiums than if the insurance had been purchased independently. A major factor in the cost of the health insurance premiums in each state will depend on the number of individuals participating in the marketplace. Thus, enrolling as many eligible individuals as possible is critically important for the overall success of the ACA.

As previously stated, the Medicaid expansion provisions of the ACA can benefit as many as 32 million enrollees. However, the reluctance of some states to participate in the ACA Medicaid expansion, the lack of public knowledge about the actual benefits of the ACA at the state level, and the sheer numbers of uninsured Americans make the enrollment process challenging. Although the framers of ACA did not foresee the Supreme Court's decision to make Medicaid expansion optional for states, the legislation did anticipate other barriers to full enrollment when the law was drafted. Consequently, the ACA provides "navigators" to conduct community outreach, education, and enrollment assistance to eligible individuals, particularly those from racial and ethnic communities and those with limited

English proficiency. The navigators must communicate effectively with those interested in enrolling in their preferred language and in a culturally competent manner. The ACA will also provide assistance to help enrollees with their applications to determine Medicaid eligibility as well as selecting the health and behavioral health services provider that will best meet their needs.

In terms of health insurance reform, the ACA makes insurance available to those who were previously excluded due to preexisting conditions. Understandably, many individuals from racial and ethnic communities have preexisting conditions due to their lack of insurance coverage and participation in the larger health care system. In addition to forbidding the denial of insurance coverage based on a preexisting health condition, the ACA allows youth to keep or obtain and maintain insurance coverage under their parents' policy up to the age of 26, a provision that has already resulted in coverage for as many as 3.1 million additional young adults (U.S. Department of Health and Human Services, 2012).

As previously mentioned, the ACA helps create new entities in each state, known as health insurance exchanges or health insurance "marketplaces" to assist enrollees to find the health insurance plan best suited for them. At present, 18 states have chosen to establish their own marketplaces. The federal government will establish marketplaces for states that fail to do so on their own. States have the option of developing a marketplace in partnership with the federal government, a choice made by six states at this time. Each state's health insurance marketplace will provide comparative analyses of available insurance plans that individuals or small employers can purchase. This "one-stop shop" will help enrollees understand the coverage available for their specific health conditions and assist them in making informed health care insurance purchasing decisions.

## CONCLUSION

The lack of health insurance negatively affects the quality of life of all Americans, whether they live in the community or in some type of institution. However, this lack of health care insurance especially impacts individuals from racial and ethnic minority communities with chronic, yet in some instances, preventable health conditions. The ACA will increase access to insurance coverage for 32 million Americans, about half of whom are from racial and ethnic minority communities. It also calls for an expansion of preventive health care, health promotion, and integration of primary and behavioral health care. The ACA seeks to address health care disparities through a focus on cultural and linguistic competence of providers and increased research on the development of evidence-based practices and supports. The ACA also calls for an increase in the number and diversity of a culturally competent health care workforce. The ACA is a historic step forward in providing equal access and health equity to racial and ethnic communities. It represents one of the greatest advances in public financing of health care since the enactment of Medicare and Medicaid in 1965 (Center for Medicare Advocacy, 2013).

The ACA recognizes that the health and well-being of all Americans requires more than access to affordable health care. Addressing the social determinants of health is key to the reduction of health disparities among racial and ethnic minority populations. The ACA provides opportunities for addressing social determinants and laying the groundwork for exploring meaningful policies and reforms that will change and improve the quality of life in every community. Dr. Adewale Troutman, President of the American Public Health Association, recently summed up the need to confront the social determinants of health in our society in this statement: "We must build on the moral imperative for addressing the social determinants of health and we must recognize that we need a long-term sustained involvement of multiple sectors that influence them" (Troutman, 2013, p. 3).

Currently 26 states will not fully implement the ACA. This decision places millions of Americans in jeopardy of not having access to affordable and needed health care. Furthermore, many individuals in these and other states might not have received the necessary information to fully understand the health benefits provided through the ACA. As a result of the lack of information and misunderstanding, many individuals may be reluctant to enroll or not know how to enroll through employers and the health insurance exchange marketplaces. A concerted effort by community leaders, service providers, legislators, health and behavioral health care consumers, and other stakeholders is needed to enroll every eligible person in the ACA. Through the effective implementation of the ACA, more racial and ethnic minority populations will gain access to quality health care services and reduce health disparities. When that occurs, people of color will experience health equity and health as a right—and so will the rest of America.

## REFERENCES

Alonso-Zaldivar, R. (2013, May 26). Republicans: Obamacare is key to 2014. *Huffington Post*. Retrieved from http://www.huffingtonpost.com/2013/05/26/republicans-obamacare_n_3339853.html?utm_hp_ref=maghreb

Bowen, S., & Canada, C. H. (2001). *Language barriers in access to health care*. Retrieved from http://www.hc-sc.gc.ca/hcs-sss/pubs/acces/2001-lang-acces/index-eng.php

Center for Medicare Advocacy. (2013). *Medicare's future: Letting the Affordable Care Act work, while learning from the past*. Willimantic, CT: Author. Retrieved from http://www.medicareadvocacy.org/medicares-future-letting-the-affordable-care-act-work-while-learning-from-the-past/

Centers for Disease Control and Prevention. (2013). Adverse Childhood Experiences (ACE) Study. Retrieved from http://www.cdc.gov/ace/

Centers for Medicare and Medicaid Services. (2013). Program of All-Inclusive Care for the Elderly. Retrieved from http://www.medicaid.gov/Medicaid-CHIP-Program-Information/By-Topics/Long-Term-Services-and-Support/Integrating-Care/Program-of-All-Inclusive-Care-for-the-Elderly-PACE/Program-of-All-Inclusive-Care-for-the-Elderly-PACE.html

CNN. (2008, August 13). Minorities expected to be majority in 2050. Retrieved from http://www.cnn.com/2008/US/08/13/census.minorities/index.html?iref=story-search

DeJongh, J. P. (2010). Implementing health care reform. Retrieved from http://www.governordejongh.com/healthreform/questions-answers/index.html

Glaze, L. (2011). *Bulletin: Correctional population in the United States, 2010.* Washington, DC: Bureau of Justice Statistics, U.S. Department of Justice. Retrieved from http://bjs.ojp.usdoj.gov/content/pub/pdf/cpus10.pdf

Hirth, V., Baskins, J., & Dever-Bumba, M. (2009). Program of All-Inclusive Care (PACE): Past, present, and future. *Journal of the American Medical Directors Association, 10*, 155–160. Retrieved from http://www.dhcs.ca.gov/provgovpart/Documents/Waiver%20Renewal/PACE_Article_JAMDA_091.pdf

Holahan, J., Buettgens, M., Carroll, C., & Dorn, S. (2012). *The cost and coverage implications of the ACA Medicaid expansion: National and state-by-state analysis.* Washington, DC: The Kaiser Family Foundation. Retrieved from http://kaiserfamilyfoundation.files.wordpress.com/2013/01/8384.pdf

Kaiser Commission on Medicaid and the Uninsured. (2013). *Impact of the Medicaid expansion for low-income communities of color across states.* Washington, DC: The Kaiser Family Foundation. Retrieved from http://kaiserfamilyfoundation.files.wordpress.com/2013/04/8435.pdf

Kaiser Family Foundation. (2013). *Status of state action on the Medicaid expansion decision, 2014.* Washington, DC: Author. Retrieved from http://kff.org/medicaid/state-indicator/state-activity-around-expanding-medicaid-under-the-affordable-care-act/#map

Kerby, S. (2012, March 17). 1 in 3 black men go to prison? The 10 most disturbing facts about racial inequality in the U.S. Criminal Justice System. *The American Prospect.* Retrieved from http://www.alternet.org/module/printversion/154587

Kurtz, A. (2013). White kids will no longer be a majority in just a few years. *CNN Money.* Retrieved from http://money.cnn.com/2013/05/15/news/economy/minority-majority/index.html

Pacific Island Health Officers' Association. (2013). About PIHOA. Retrieved from http://pihoa.org/about/index.php

Pernas, I. (2012). *Impact of federal health reform in the quality of healthcare in Puerto Rico: A multi-sector perspective.* Guaynabo, PR: Pharmaceutical Industry Association of Puerto Rico. Retrieved from http://www.piapr.org/clientuploads/5th%20Market%20Access%20Summit%20PP%20%28Sept.14,%202012%29/Lcda%20Iraelia%20Pernas.pdf

Pew Research Center. (2011). *Minorities account for nearly all U.S. population growth.* Retrieved from http://www.pewresearch.org/daily-number/minorities-account-for-nearly-all-u-s-population-growth/

Phillips, S. (2012). *The Affordable Care Act: Implications for public safety and corrections populations*. Washington, DC: The Sentencing Project. Retrieved from http://www.sentencingproject.org/doc/publications/inc_Affordable_Care_Act.pdf

Smedley, B., Stith, A., & Nelson, A. (2003). *Unequal treatment: Confronting racial and ethnic disparities in health care*. Washington, DC: National Academies Press. Retrieved from http://www.iom.edu/Reports/2002/Unequal-Treatment-Confronting-Racial-and-Ethnic-Disparities-in-Health-Care.aspx

Thomas, M., & James, C. (2009). *The role of health coverage for communities of color*. Washington, DC: The Kaiser Family Foundation. Retrieved from http://kaiserfamilyfoundation.files.wordpress.com/2013/01/8017.pdf

Troutman, A. (2013). Turning our growing focus on social determinants of health into practice. *The Nation's Health*, *43*(5), 3.

U.S. Census Bureau. (2006). *Vintage 2006: National tables*. Washington, DC: Author. Retrieved from http://www.census.gov/popest/data/historical/2000s/vintage_2006/

U.S. Department of Health and Human Services. (2012). *State-level estimates of gains in insurance coverage among young adults*. Retrieved from http://www.hhs.gov/healthcare/facts/factsheets/2012/06/young-adults06192012a.html

U.S. Virgin Islands Bureau of Economic Research. (2009). *Comprehensive economic development strategy for the United States Virgin Islands 2009*. Washington, DC: U.S. Department of the Interior. Retrieved from http://www.doi.gov/oia/reports/upload/USVI-CEDS-2009-2.pdf

# Overview of the Affordable Care Act's Impact on Military and Veteran Mental Health Services: Nine Implications for Significant Improvements in Care

MARK C. RUSSELL

*Institute of War Stress Injury, Recovery, & Social Justice, Antioch University Seattle, Seattle, Washington, USA*

CHARLES R. FIGLEY

*Tulane Traumatology Institute, Tulane University, New Orleans, Louisiana, USA*

*On March 23, 2010, President Barack Obama signed the Affordable Care Act (ACA) into law. Implications of the ACA on mental health care for 9.7 million military active-duty, reserve, and family members and 22.2 million veterans, as well as 1.3 uninsured veterans, is reviewed in light of a major crisis. The authors trace historical roots of the ACA to the World War II generation and efforts to transform the mental health care system by implementing hard-won war trauma lessons. The authors posit 9 principles reflected in the ACA that represent unfulfilled generational war trauma lessons and potential transformation of the military and national mental health care systems.*

Each moment of combat imposes a strain so great that men will break down in direct relation to the intensity and duration of their exposure. Thus psychiatric casualties are as inevitable as gunshot and shrapnel wounds in warfare.

—Appel and Beebe (1946, p. 185)

By 2014, the United States plans to end its longest war. In its wake, a major wartime behavioral health crisis unfolds as 100,000 to 150,000 of more than 2.6 million war veterans transition out of the military each year, along with skyrocketing individual and financial costs associated with escalating prevalence of war stress injuries such as posttraumatic stress disorder (PTSD), depression, suicide, substance abuse, traumatic grief, military sexual trauma, posttraumatic anger, traumatic brain injury (TBI), and medically unexplained physical symptoms (MUPS).

On March 23, 2010, President Barack Obama signed H.R. 3590, the Patient Protection and Affordable Care Act (commonly called the Affordable Care Act [ACA]), but also referred to as the Health Care Reform Act (HCRA), into law as Public Law 111-148, making it the law of the land. The controversial insurance mandate of ACA is essential in overhauling a $2.7 trillion health care system and proximate universal health coverage, most of which takes effect the same year U.S. troops are expected to leave Afghanistan in 2014 (Patient Protection and Affordable Care Act, 2010, Veteran's Administration, 2010). Jaffe (2012) analyzed the historic U.S. Supreme Court decision that settled a contentious legal debate over sweeping health care reforms that offer coverage to some 30 million uninsured Americans (e.g., Congressional Budget Office [CBO], 2012). In return for gaining a heftier pool of beneficiaries, insurers are now prohibited from charging higher insurance rates for women or for beneficiaries with preexisting conditions and cannot refuse or terminate coverage (Jaffe, 2012).

Per the ACA, beginning in 2014, individuals without health insurance will face an initial tax penalty of $95 that grows to $695 in 2016 and increases annually with cost-of-living adjustments (Jaffe, 2012). Before and after passage of the ACA, a frenzy of confusion, contradictory messages, and misinformation ensued, especially in regard to its potential negative impact within military populations. A variety of political leaders, news media, and veterans' support organizations raised fears about abandoning returning war veterans in their time of need (Maze, 2009). A particular concern to the estimated 14 million beneficiaries of the health care programs in the Department of Defense (DoD) and the Department of Veterans Health Affairs (VA), providing insurance at a combined cost in 2011 of $104 billion (TRICARE, 2012a), centered around escalating health care costs and reductions in hard-earned benefits. Now that much of the dust has cleared, what, if any effect will the ACA actually have on the military population, particularly in regard to mental health services during a time of crisis?

In this article, we examine how ACA implementation will affect military populations and the mental health services they can expect to receive in the immediate and distant future. First we briefly review the historical context for judging the ACA in light of wartime behavioral health.

## HISTORICAL CONTEXT

A search for comparable federal health care legislation, with similar potential to transform the American mental health landscape, harkens back to 1945 and the ending of World War II (1939–1945). As post–World War II American society struggled with the fallout from its own wartime behavioral health crisis resulting from a reported 1.3 million military neuropsychiatric admissions, with more than 600,000 psychiatrically discharged veterans rapidly overwhelming a completely inept VA system (Baker & Pickren, 2007), legends of enlightened former military leaders became disillusioned with the fragmented, antiquated, dualistic mental health care policies in the private sector that emphasized social isolation, stigma, and institutionalization (Menninger, 1948). Specifically, crucial paradigmatic changes gleaned from hard-won psychiatric lessons of World War II were tragically being ignored in the public sector. This new military paradigm centered on the treatability of traumatic stress injuries and the need for a coordinated continuum of holistic care focusing on prevention, early identification, and intervention, as well as critical social reintegration services with clear expectations of recovery, along well-defined, integrated echelons of community-based treatment aimed to support families and restore the individual to a maximal level of functioning and productivity (Glass & Bernucci, 1966). These seasoned clinicians also knew that changing hearts and minds would require a concerted effort and resources to generate the necessary public awareness, destigmatization, and social reintegration implemented by well-trained, knowledgeable practitioners—informed by scientific investigation and innovation (Menninger, 1948). A large cadre of such leaders was all too familiar with the perilous consequences of neglecting so-called psychiatric lessons of war (Jones, 1995), resulting in many becoming staunch reform advocates (e.g., Glass, 1966; Menninger, 1948).

Consequently, on July 3, 1946, H.R. 2550, the prodigiously bipartisan National Neuropsychiatric Institute Act, was signed by President Harry S. Truman into public law as the National Mental Health Act (Grob & Goldman, 2006). This key piece of legislation created the National Institute of Mental Health (NIMH), intended to reposition mental health on par with physical health, and close the research, public education, treatment, and policy chasm between the medical and psychological sciences (Grob & Goldman, 2006). In 1955, the Korean War (1950–1953) armistice was signed and Congress passed the Mental Health Study Act, establishing the Joint Commission on Mental Illness and Health (JCMIH; Grob & Goldman, 2006). The JCMIH was a first of its kind, congressionally funded multidisciplinary team of national experts and leaders from the NIMH, American Psychiatric Association, American Medical Association, Council of State Governments, representatives from clinical psychology, psychiatric social work, nursing, and the Veterans Administration (Grob & Goldman, 2006). The JCMIH mandate was essentially to design an integrated comprehensive mental health system based on many of the psychiatric lessons born of war. In particular, the JCMIH was tasked with the following:

1. To study the biopsychosocial and cultural etiological factors of mental illness.
2. To identify, develop, and apply appropriate assessment, diagnosis, treatment, and rehabilitation services.
3. To evaluate the recruitment and training of mental health personnel.
4. To conduct a national survey of mental health care to help design a comprehensive program.
5. To widely disseminate the reported findings and public education (Grob & Goldman, 2006).

In 1961, the JCMIH's final report, *Action for Mental Health* was submitted to Congress, state governors, and the general public, recommending a comprehensive integrated national program made up of four interrelated elements:

1. Greater investment in basic research to reduce the gap in scientific knowledge.
2. Adoption of national recruitment and training programs to increase the supply of well-trained mental health clinicians who would provide an integrated, continuum (echelon) of community-based mental health services reflecting previous wartime experiences.
3. A pressing need to destigmatize mental health needs by a national public education campaign.
4. A dramatic and progressive increase in federal funding of mental health resources to raise standards of care (Grob & Goldman, 2006).

Unfortunately, political in-fighting among health care stakeholders and government officials resulted in greatly watered-down legislation. In 1963, President John F. Kennedy signed the Mental Retardation and Community Mental Health Centers Construction Act that eventually would lead to deinstitutionalization and community mental health programs. However, many wartime lessons were tragically ignored (e.g., adequate resourcing, ending stigma and disparity, etc.).

Since 1963, every subsequent piece of mental health legislation has fallen critically short of realizing the transformative reforms envisioned in 1945 and 1961, until the 2008 enactment of the Mental Health Parity and Addiction Equity Act (Grob & Goldman, 2006). This law's passage constituted a key first step toward ending the disparity in caring for people with mental health and addiction disorders by requiring parity in coverage equal to medical and surgical benefits. The subsequent passing of the ACA 2 years later marks the continuation of a nation still struggling to awaken to the realities of mental health and honor its lessons of war trauma. Nevertheless, despite well-documented psychiatric lessons since World War I (1914–1918), and particularly those relearned and learned during World War II (Glass, 1966), the U.S. military has consistently ignored these lessons, resulting in behavioral health crises after every subsequent war up to the present date (M. C. Russell & Figley, 2013).

In short, both civilian and military U.S. mental health systems continue to be plagued by antiquated, dualistic health care practices; contradictory, ambiguous, and fragmented policies and organizations; reliably poor planning and preparation; and chronic and severe underresourcing, including ominous shortages of well-trained personnel, all of which reinforce disparity, stigma, and barriers to care that perpetuate cyclic crises (e.g., Department of Defense Task Force on Mental Health, 2007; M. C. Russell & Figley, 2013).

## POTENTIAL POSITIVE IMPACT OF THE ACA ON AMERICAN MENTAL HEALTH CARE

There are many "new" and noteworthy implications of the ACA. First, and foremost, the ACA establishes the precedent that all Americans, regardless of race, ethnicity, gender, age, socioeconomic status, or type of illness, have a basic right to access quality health care including mental health services. According to Cabaj (2011), beginning on September 23, 2010, many key ACA provisions have already been activated that strengthen consumer protection and limit abuse by insurance companies including the following:

- Young people up to age 26 are able to remain on their parents' insurance policies.
- Insurers are prohibited from denying coverage to children with preexisting conditions.
- Insurers are no longer able to cancel individuals' policies except in cases of outright consumer fraud.
- Lifetime limits (limits on the amount of money insurers will pay in claims over an individual's lifetime) are prohibited.
- New restrictions are placed on insurers' ability to impose annual limits.
- Insurance plans are required to cover certain preventive services, including depression screening and regular behavioral assessments for children.

## DIFFERENTIAL IMPACTS OF THE ACA

To understand the potential impact of the ACA on military populations, it is crucial to differentiate the various military-related subcomponents, as each

THE AFFORDABLE CARE ACT AND INTEGRATED BEHAVIORAL HEALTH CARE

group has unique health care plans and different access to mental health services. The military population includes the active-duty service component (Air Force, Army, Marine Corps, and Navy), the active Reserve and National Guard component, DoD civilians (federal employees and contractors), military retirees, "veterans" eligible for VA care, family members, and former military personnel and "uninsured veterans" ineligible for VA care. The term *veteran* can be confusing. It is often used interchangeably for describing active-duty personnel returning from war, any individual who has served in the military (active duty or reserve component), and only discharged military members who are war veterans. The later designation is what we adhere to here.

## Active Duty Component

According to the Defense Manpower Data Center (2010), of the total of 1,414,951 active-duty personnel in the DoD, 1,212,228 (86%) are male, and 202,723 (14%) are female. The total number of enlisted active-duty members is 1,184,002, with 1,017,201 male and 166,801 female. In contrast, there are only 211,741 officers in the DoD, of whom 177,403 are male, and 34,338 are female, and an additional total of 19,208 warrant officers. Overall, approximately 33% of active duty and 25% of reserves are racial or ethnic minorities (Defense Manpower Data Center, 2010). In 2006, almost half of the active component enlisted members were between the ages of 17 and 24 years old, compared to approximately 14% of the comparable civilian labor force matched for age (Office of the Under Secretary of Defense, Personnel, and Readiness, 2006). Approximately 56% of active-duty personnel are married, including 541,445 active-duty members single without children, and another 75,000 who are single parents. There are approximately 94,890 joint service marriages, and 702,716 service members are married to a civilian (Defense Manpower Data Center, 2010). All active-duty personnel are automatically enrolled in TRICARE Prime, and family members and retirees under 65 years old have the option of choosing from TRICARE Prime, TRICARE Extra, and TRICARE Standard (TRICARE, 2012a).

## Active Reserve

Active Reserve and National Guard personnel make up the Reserve Component (RC) that serves as an "auxiliary" or augmenting force to the active-duty component in times of state or national urgency (Best, 2007). The RC troops have been deployed in greater numbers than at any time in recent history, constituting 38% to 40% or more of the deployed force. The active Reserve is distinguished from the inactive Reserve, who are former military personnel without any obligated active reserve service, subject to recall only via presidential order. National Guard subcomponents consist of the Army National

Guard, Army Reserve, Navy Reserve, Marine Reserve, Air National Guard, and the Air Force Reserve. Length of time that the RC may be mobilized or activated to active-duty status depends on the nature of the mission (i.e., disaster or humanitarian relief, wartime deployment), which can vary from months to 1 year.

According to the Defense Manpower Data Center (2010), the total number of the RC is 852,290 personnel, 82% of whom are male, and 18% female. Overall, approximately 25% of the RC are racial or ethnic minorities with 14.7% Black, 69% White, 0.9% Native American, 2.7% Asian, and 9.3% Hispanic (Defense Manpower Data Center, 2010). Nearly 32% of the RC enlisted members are between the ages of 17 and 24 years old compared to approximately 14% of the comparable civilian labor force matched for age (Office of the Under Secretary of Defense, Personnel, and Readiness, 2006).

HEALTH CARE BENEFITS

All National Guard and other RC members are automatically enrolled in TRICARE Prime and might also be eligible for VA health care if they were called to active duty by a federal order and completed the full period for which they were called (TRICARE, 2012a). TRICARE provides a broad array of benefits coverage for RC members and their families, from predeployment and during mobilization, to postdeployment and into retirement from the Selected Reserves (TRICARE, 2012a).

RC members and their families receive premium-free TRICARE coverage for up to 180 days before the sponsor reports for active duty in support of a named contingency operation (early eligibility), and for 180 days after deactivation through the Transitional Assistance Management Program (TAMP; TRICARE, 2012a). The premium-based TRICARE Reserve Select (TRS) health plan offers comprehensive services and TRICARE Standard and TRICARE Extra coverage was established by the 2005 National Defense Authorization Act (NDAA) for qualified members of the Selected Reserves and their immediate family members (*Federal Register,* March 5, 2005, cited in TRICARE, 2012a). The number of plans (member-only and family) and number of covered lives have increased sixfold since the October 2007 changes, from almost 12,000 plans and 35,000 covered lives beginning in FY 2008, to over 76,000 plans and 201,000 covered lives by the end of FY 2011 (TRICARE, 2012a). TRS monthly premiums changed from FY 2011 to FY 2012 as follows: TRS member only $53.16 to $54.35; TRS member and family $197.76 to $192.89 (see www.tricare.mil/trs, cited in TRICARE, 2012a).

Coverage under the TRICARE Retired Reserve (TRR) premium-based health plan began on October 1, 2010, in response to the NDAA for FY 2010, Section 705 and Title 10 United States Code, Chapter 55, Section 1076e (cited in TRICARE, 2012a). The law allows qualified members of the

Retired Reserve to purchase full-cost premium-based coverage under TRR until they reach age 60, when they receive premium-free TRICARE coverage for themselves as retirees and their eligible family members (TRICARE, 2012a). TRR premiums changed from FY 2011 to FY 2012 as follows: TRR member only $408.01 to $419.72; TRR member and family $1,020.05 to $1,024.43 (www.tricare.mil/trs, cited in TRICARE, 2012a).

## DoD Civilian Employees

There are approximately 779,163 full-time, DoD civilian federal employees and an unknown number of civilian contractors and local civilian hires (Defense Manpower Data Center, 2010).

### HEALTH CARE BENEFITS

The Federal Employee Health Benefits Program (FEHBP) was established by law in 1959 and became active in 1960 (Office of Personnel Management [OPM], 2009). It is administered by the OPM and provides federal employees and eligible family members with a variety of privately run, government-subsidized insurance plans. Among the plan types are fee-for-service (FFS) plans, high-deductible health plans, and health maintenance organization (HMO) plans (OPM, 2009). Plans may not turn down employees or eligible family members because of preexisting medical conditions (OPM, 2009). In general, costs of the plan are split between the employee and the federal government: The government pays the smaller of 75% of the chosen plan cost or 72% of the average plan cost of all FEHBP enrollees (OPM, 2009). Most federal employees are eligible for the FEHBP. On retirement, qualified employees may continue enrollment in their current plan (OPM, 2009). The mental health services and providers covered by the plans differ by care organization, options purchased, and the state in which the plan was purchased, and may vary year to year (OPM, 2009). There are no known changes from the ACA impacting DoD civilian employees and FEHBP, and therefore we exclude them from further analysis.

## Military Retirees

Active-duty personnel are eligible to retire after 20 to 30 years of military service, wherein they receive a monthly pension adjusted by their rank, years of service, and year of entry. However, 83% of service members do not retire from the military. In FY 2011, TRICARE provided coverage to 3.08 million eligible retirees and family members under the age of 65 years (34%) and 1.92 million eligible retirees and family members over the age of 65 years (21%; TRICARE, 2012a). Retirees might or might not be "veterans" in the sense of having deployed to a war zone, and might not be eligible to receive mental health care benefits through the VA if they had no documented disability from a mental health condition while on active duty. In those cases, retirees will likely utilize TRICARE, private insurance, or both (TRICARE, 2012b). A percentage of retirees will also be eligible for both VA and TRICARE mental health benefits (TRICARE, 2012a).

HEALTH CARE BENEFITS

All military retirees under 65 years old have the option of choosing from TRICARE Prime, TRICARE Extra, and TRICARE Standard (TRICARE, 2012a). Between FY 2001 and FY 2011, 23.8% of retirees switched from private health insurance to TRICARE (TRICARE, 2012a). Most of these retirees likely switched because of the increasing disparity in premiums (and out-of-pocket expenses); in the past few years, some might have lost coverage due to the recession. As a result of declines in private insurance coverage, an additional 732,000 retirees and family members under age 65 are now relying primarily on TRICARE instead of private health insurance (TRICARE, 2012a). If eligible military retirees who are war veterans or have been diagnosed with a service-connected mental health condition, they may also utilize VA mental health care (TRICARE, 2012b).

## Veterans and Eligibility for VA Mental Health Benefits

As of September 30, 2011, there were an estimated 22.2 million living veterans (Government Accountability Office [GAO], 2011b). The term *veteran* typically refers to military personnel who have deployed to a war zone. As of March 2010, more than 60% of all veterans were 55 years of age or older. Female veterans are a growing demographic in the veteran population—from FY 2010 to FY 2020 the percentage of female veterans in the total veteran population is projected to increase from approximately 8% to approximately 10% (GAO, 2011b). In November 2010, Reservists and National Guard members made up nearly 50% of the Operation Enduring Freedom (OEF)/Operation Iraqi Freedom (OIF) veteran population (GAO, 2011b). According to the GAO (2011b), the VA's Office of Rural Health reported that in FY 2010, 41% of veterans enrolled in the VA lived in rural areas.

The VA manages access to services in relation to available resources through a priority system established by law. Panangala (2010) explained that the order of VA priorities is mostly determined by service-connected disability, income, or other special status such as the following:

- Those given honorable discharges qualify for VA health care if they are low-income; the threshold is $30,460 a year for a single veteran with no dependents. A veteran with five dependents gets health care if he or she makes less than $45,000.

THE AFFORDABLE CARE ACT AND INTEGRATED BEHAVIORAL HEALTH CARE

- The VA provides 5 years of cost-free health care to Iraq and Afghanistan veterans for any injury or illness associated with their service.
- Beyond that, veterans get VA medical care with varying copayment levels if they were injured during their service or if an illness is judged to be service connected.
- A veteran held as a prisoner of war or who is a Purple Heart medal recipient is eligible. So is a veteran who receives a VA pension or disability benefits.
- Additionally, Congress has stipulated that certain combat veterans discharged from active duty on or after January 2003 are eligible for priority enrollment (GAO, 2011b).

HEALTH CARE BENEFITS

In general, veterans must enroll in VA health care to receive VA's mental health benefits, which include a full range of hospital and outpatient services, prescription drugs, and noninstitutional long-term care services. There are essentially three categories of insurance plans for veterans. According to Kizer (2012), the majority (56%) have private health insurance or are covered by a non-VA health plan. Thirty-seven percent receive health care services through the VA health care system, which bases eligibility on having a service-connected disability (SCD), low income level and net worth, or other specific circumstances. More than 80% of VA enrollees older than 65 years also are covered by Medicare, and about 25% are beneficiaries of two or more non-VA federal health plans, such as Medicare, Medicaid, TRICARE, or Indian Health Service. Seven percent of veterans have no health insurance (Kizer, 2012).

COST-SHARING RULES

The VA provides treatment for SCDs free of charge to all enrolled veterans. Veterans in the highest priority groups generally do not pay inpatient or outpatient copayments even for care unrelated to their service. Copayments for outpatient services for veterans in the lower priority groups are $15 for a primary care visit and $50 for a visit to a specialist (CBO, 2007). The copayment for inpatient services for the first 90 days of care during a 365-day period is $992, and $496 for each additional 90 days of care during a 365-day period. The per diem charge for inpatient services is $10 (CBO, 2007). Those copayment rates may be reduced by 80% for veterans with income or net worth below the Department of Housing and Urban Development's geographic index (CBO, 2007). Copayments for medications are waived for veterans with very low income and those with SCD ratings of 50% or higher (CBO, 2007).

## Family Members

In FY 2011, TRICARE (2012a) reports providing coverage for 1.91 million active duty family members (21% of the total beneficiaries) and 0.55 million

National Guard and active Reserve family members (6% of total beneficiaries), as well as a large number of family members of retired personnel (see military retirees, previously discussed).

### HEALTH CARE BENEFITS

All spouses, children under the age of 21 years, and dependent adults of an active-duty, active Reserve and National Guard, military retiree, or survivor of a deceased war veteran or retiree, have the option of choosing from TRICARE Prime, TRICARE Extra, and TRICARE Standard (TRICARE, 2012a). Family members are generally ineligible for VA mental health care, except those specialized programs for family members. Family members of former military personnel who did not retire or die from military service, or were diagnosed with an SCD, are typically ineligible for TRICARE and VA coverage, and thus are "uninsured" (TRICARE, 2012a). There are an estimated 950,000 uninsured family members of veterans who report significantly less access to needed health care than their counterparts with insurance coverage (U.S. Census Bureau, 2012).

## Former Military Personnel and Uninsured Veterans

According to the U.S. Census Bureau (2012), a recent American Community Survey (ACS) revealed that 1 in 10 of 12.5 million nonelderly veterans (19–64 years old) reported being uninsured and ineligible for VA health care. Age aside, there are an estimated 1.3 million uninsured veterans nationwide, with another 0.9 million veterans using VA care, but without other health insurance coverage, and an additional 0.9 million uninsured family members (U.S. Census Bureau, 2012). More than 40% of uninsured veterans report having unmet medical needs, and about a third have delayed care due to costs (Hayley & Kenney, 2012).

### HEALTH BENEFITS

A large segment of the active-duty, Reserve, and National Guard components do not retire from the military, and instead, they either complete their period of obligated service honorably (e.g., 4-year enlistment contract) or are administratively separated from the military for cause (e.g., misconduct, rehab failure, personality disorder), and are thus generally ineligible for further health care benefits from either TRICARE or VA. An exception would be those former military personnel who are eligible to receive VA mental health care due to a diagnosed service-connected mental health condition (e.g., PTSD). Hayley and Kenney (2012) reported that uninsured veterans and family members indicated significantly less access to essential health care than their insured counterparts. A comparative analysis of insured and uninsured veterans revealed that uninsured vets served more recently, are younger, are more likely to be single, have lower education levels, and are more likely to be unemployed than insured veterans (U.S. Census Bureau, 2010). Consequently, uninsured veterans and their family members have less access to employer-sponsored insurance coverage (Hayley & Kenney, 2012).

## OVERVIEW OF THE MILITARY HEALTH CARE SYSTEM

The Military Health System (MHS) is a global medical network within the DoD responsible for providing health care to 9.7 million beneficiaries who include active-duty, reservists, National Guard, retirees, family members, survivors, and certain former spouses worldwide (MHS, 2012). The primary mission of the MHS is to maintain the health and readiness of military personnel, so they can carry out their military missions, and to be prepared to deliver health care required during wartime (MHS, 2012). As of 2012, the MHS is equipped with 56 (41 in the United States) military treatment facilities (MTFs), 365 (293 in the United States) outpatient health clinics, and employs 144,376 medical personnel (86,007 enlisted and officers, and 58,369 DoD civilians; TRICARE, 2012a).

TRICARE is the MHS health care benefits program for all seven uniformed services—the Army, the Navy, the Marine Corps, the Air Force, the Coast Guard, the Commissioned Corps of the Public Health Service, and the Commissioned Corps of the National Oceanic and Atmospheric Administration—and the National Guard and Reserves. According to the Institutes of Medicine (IOM, 2010), TRICARE represents a continuation of a national commitment to provide quality health care for military populations that began in 1775. The TRICARE Management Activity (TMA) under the DoD Assistant Secretary of Defense for Health Affairs (civilian head, MHS) manages TRICARE by organizing into six geographic health service regions (MHS, 2012). In addition, TRICARE's civilian Purchased Care Systems is made up of a network of 438,424 individual providers (primary care, behavioral health, and specialty care providers), 59,587 of whom are behavioral (mental) health providers (MHS, 2012).

## Eligible Beneficiaries

In FY 2011, TRICARE served 9.72 million active duty, National Guard, and Reserve members, retirees, their families, and survivors worldwide, up from 9.59 million in FY 2009 (MHS, 2012). A total of 9.11 million (94%) were stationed or resided in the United States and 0.60 million were stationed or resided abroad (TRICARE, 2012a). The number of enrolled beneficiaries remained at about 5.5 million from FY 2009 to FY 2011. The Army has the most beneficiaries eligible for Uniformed Services health care benefits, followed (in order) by the Air Force, Navy, Marine Corps, and other Uniformed Services (TRICARE, 2012a). Whereas retirees and their family members constitute the largest percentage of the eligible population (55%) in the United States, active duty personnel (including Guard/RC members on active duty for at least 30 days) and their family members make up the largest percentage (68%) of the eligible population abroad (TRICARE, 2012a).

## Estimated Cost of Mental Health Care in Military Populations

The combined costs for DoD and VA health care in FY 2011 were $104 billion, or about 11% of all federal health expenditures (Merlis, 2012). In regard to the MHS, $54 billion slated for the Unified Medical Program (UMP) for FY 2012 is 16% greater than the almost $47 billion spent in FY 2009 (cited in TRICARE, 2012a). The UMP was 5.4% of the FY 2011 total defense expenditures (including the normal cost contribution to the Accrual Fund for retirees), and was expected to be almost 7% of the FY 2012 defense budget as currently programmed (TRICARE, 2012a). Specific to mental health care, MHS expenditures on TBI and psychological health conditions were $417 million in FY 2008, $533 million in FY 2009, $578 million in FY 2010, and $669 million in FY 2011 (TRICARE, 2012a, p. 18).

The VA spent an estimated $52 billion providing medical care to veterans in 2012, or 40% of the Department of Veterans Affairs total budget (Merlis, 2012). In regard to VA mental health care expenditures, studies estimated that costs associated with PTSD for Iraq and Afghanistan ranged from $708 million to $1.2 billion, translating into a cost per patient of $5,904 to $10,298 in the 2 years after discharge from the military (IOM, 2012). According to the IOM (2012), in FY 2010, the VA spent $112,460,032 on specialized outpatient PTSD programs, treating 105,531 veterans, for an average of 10 visits per year, costing $1,066 per veteran (or $105 per session). The VA also spent $42,716,581 on 5,128 admissions to specialized intensive PTSD programs in FY 2010, averaging $8,330 per veteran (IOM, 2012).

## TRICARE Health Plan Options

Military populations enrolled in TRICARE have several options in terms of insurance coverage. The following brief summaries are from TRICARE (2012a).

### TRICARE PRIME

This is the HMO-like benefit offered in many areas. Each enrollee chooses or is assigned a primary care manager (PCM), a health care professional who is responsible for helping the patient manage his or her care, promoting preventive health services (e.g., routine exams, immunizations), and arranging for specialty provider services as appropriate. Access standards apply to waiting times to get an appointment and waiting times in doctors' offices. A point-of-service (POS) option permits enrollees to seek care from providers other than the assigned PCM without a referral, but with significantly higher deductibles and cost shares.

### TRICARE STANDARD

The nonnetwork benefit, formerly known as the Civilian Health and Medical Program of the Uniformed Services (CHAMPUS), is open to all eligible DoD beneficiaries, except active duty service members (ADSMs). Beneficiaries who are eligible for Medicare Part B are also covered by TRICARE Standard for any services covered by TRICARE but not covered by Medicare. Once eligibility is recorded in the Defense Enrollment Eligibility Reporting System (DEERS), no further application is required from beneficiaries to obtain care from TRICARE-authorized civilian providers. An annual deductible (individual or family) and cost shares are required.

### TRICARE EXTRA

This is the network benefit for beneficiaries eligible for TRICARE Standard. When nonenrolled beneficiaries obtain services from TRICARE network professionals, hospitals, and suppliers, they pay the same deductible as TRICARE Standard; however, TRICARE Extra cost shares are reduced by 5%. TRICARE network providers file claims for the beneficiary.

### TRICARE FOR LIFE

This is the Defense Authorization Act for FY 2001 (Pub, L. 106-259) to serve as a second payer to Medicare for retirees for TRICARE beneficiaries 65 years old and older who are entitled to Medicare Part A and enrolled in Medicare Part B; it offers full coverage for many services only partially covered by Medicare. Congress also extended a pharmacy benefit to Medicare-eligible beneficiaries.

## Military Mental Health Care Services

Mental health services are provided by the MHS through the three military medical departments (Air Force, Army, Navy [which includes Marine Corps]; TRICARE; and civilian contractors; MHS, 2012). However, each of the military branches also provides a range of mental health services outside of its respective medical departments through various family, community, and warrior support centers, as well as through the military Chaplain Corps. The organization of military mental health care services is inherently fragmented, with each military medical department assigning active-duty and DoD civilian mental health practitioners to military hospitals, referred to as MTFs, substance abuse treatment programs, or outpatient mental health clinics, which often function independently from other mental health services offered (i.e., family support centers, DoD contractors, pastoral care, etc.).

## TRICARE Covered Mental Health Services

A number of outpatient and inpatient mental health services are covered under TRICARE, such as individual, family, and group psychotherapy; psychological testing; medication management; tele-mental health program; acute inpatient psychiatric care; residential treatment; inpatient detoxification; rehabilitation; and outpatient substance use care (TRICARE, 2012b). There are limitations regarding the time, duration, or number of sessions covered per episode, admission, benefit period, or fiscal year (TRICARE, 2012b). Coverage limitations are in many cases defined by statute; specifics are in Title 10 of the USC and Title 32 of the CFR. Authorized providers recognized under TRICARE are defined in 32 CFR Part 199 and, generally, the *TRICARE Policy Manual* 6010.54-M, Chapter 11, Section 1.1. For mental health services, they include psychiatrists and other physicians, clinical psychologists, certified psychiatric nurse specialists, clinical social workers, certified marriage and family therapists, pastoral counselors, and mental health counselors (32 CFR§ 199.4(c)(3)(ix) and *TRICARE Policy Manual* 6010.54-M, Chapter 7, cited in IOM, 2010).

## TRICARE Mental Health Exclusions

The behavioral health care services not covered under TRICARE include aversion therapy; behavioral health care related solely to obesity or weight reduction; biofeedback for psychosomatic conditions; vocational counseling, and counseling for socioeconomic purposes, stress management, or lifestyle modifications; custodial nursing care; educational programs; experimental procedures; psychological testing and assessment as part of an assessment for academic placement (e.g., testing to determine whether a beneficiary has a learning disability if the primary or sole basis for the testing is to assess for a learning disability); psychosurgery; sexual dysfunction therapy; and therapy for developmental or learning disorders (TRICARE, 2012b).

## TRICARE Health Plan Costs

The maximum out-of-pocket expenses for each fiscal year (October 1–September 30) is called the *catastrophic cap*. This cap applies to annual deductibles, pharmacy copayments, TRICARE Prime enrollment fees, and all other copayments or cost shares paid for TRICARE-covered services. The cap for active duty family members is $1,000 per family, per fiscal year; for beneficiaries enrolled in TRICARE Reserve Select, it is $1,000 per family, per fiscal year; and for all others it is $3,000 per family, per fiscal year (TRICARE, 2012a).

#### COMPARISON OF OUT-OF-POCKET EXPENSES FOR FAMILIES IN TRICARE PRIME VERSUS A CIVILIAN HMO

According to the TMA, in FY 2009 through 2011, civilian counterpart families had substantially higher out-of-pocket costs than TRICARE Prime enrollees (TRICARE, 2012a). Civilian HMO counterparts paid more for insurance premiums, deductibles, and copayments. In FY 2011, costs for civilian counterparts were $4,400 more than those incurred by active-duty families enrolled in Prime and $4,100 more than those incurred by retiree families enrolled in Prime (TRICARE, 2012a).

## Deficiencies in Military Mental Health Care

A DoD Task Force on Mental Health (2007) report indicated that mental health services were generally inadequate for active-duty and RCs, and their family members due to chronic, significant underresourcing, staffing shortages, inadequate training, and dysfunctional organization. In regard to TRICARE, the Task Force concluded that "DoD's mental health providers require additional training regarding current and new state-of-the-art practice guidelines" (p. 20). The Task Force also found that there was "no consistent system for ongoing quality assessment and continuous improvement that includes substantial measurements of psychological health care outcomes" (p. 33). It concluded that "there are not sufficient mechanisms in place to assure the use of evidence-based treatments or the monitoring of treatment effectiveness" and that "the TRICARE network benefit for psychological health is hindered by fragmented rules and policies, inadequate oversight, and insufficient reimbursement" (p. ES-3).

The DoD Task Force on Mental Health (2007) also observed that several GAO investigations (GAO, 2003; U.S. Government Accountability Office, 2006) have concluded that TRICARE reimbursement rates were not competitive, resulting in providers deciding to not accept new TRICARE patients, thus further contributing to the current wartime mental health crisis. In the recent survey of TRICARE civilian providers (which did not adequately sample mental health providers), low reimbursement was the most cited reason for refusing TRICARE patients (DoD Task Force on Mental Health, 2007).

## TRANSITIONING TO THE VA HEALTH CARE SYSTEM

Another persistent concern has been continuity of care for the 100,000 to 150,000 service members each year transitioning out of the military, and possibly into the VA system. An estimated 868,000 of the 2.6 million war veterans exited the military from October 2001 through September 20, 2011, many with untreated war stress injuries such as PTSD, substance abuse, depression, and suicidal behavior (e.g., IOM, 2012). For example, Mojtabi, Rosenheck, Wyatt, and Susser (2003) reported that only 52% of transitioning military personnel discharged with severe war stress injuries (e.g., PTSD) sought VA mental health care. The National Defense Authorization Act for FY 2008 required the DoD and VA to establish a joint comprehensive care management and transition policy for military personnel recovering from a serious injury or illness, particularly those with PTSD and high suicide risk, including devising recovery plans and assigning recovery care coordinators for each service member (Merlis, 2012). Despite some positive changes, significant difficulties remain in transitioning mental health care between the DoD and the VA. Studies have indicated a number of transitioning personnel are experiencing psychological distress and that transitional services need to be alert to their psychological needs (GAO, 2011a).

## Special Eligibility Period for Combat Veterans

Traditionally, RC personnel who return from a deployment but remain on the military rolls would not qualify for VA health care until some later date when they were discharged from the service. However, legislation enacted in 1998, the Veterans Programs Enhancement Act (1998; Pub. L. 105-368), gave veterans and demobilized reservists returning from combat operations a special 2-year period of eligibility for health care from the VA, waiving any requirements for them to satisfy a means test or to demonstrate an SCD (CBO, 2007). Under that authority, the VA provides health care for free for medical conditions potentially related to military service in combat operations. In 2009, 38 U.S.C. § 1710(a), 38 C.F.R. §§ 17.36, 17.38 was passed, allowing any veteran who has served in a combat theater after November 11, 1998, including OEF/OIF veterans, and who was discharged or released from active service on or after January 28, 2003, has up to 5 years from the date of his or her most recent discharge or release from active duty service to enroll in VA's health care system and receive the VA health care services (IOM, 2012).

## OVERVIEW OF THE DEPARTMENT OF VETERANS AFFAIRS

Although its historical roots begin after the American Revolution, the establishment of the VA came in 1930 when Congress authorized the President to "consolidate and coordinate Government activities affecting war veterans" (Panangala, 2010). The VA represents the nation's largest health system, comprised of 171 medical centers; more than 350 outpatient, community, and outreach clinics; 126 nursing home care units; and 40 domiciliary (e.g., IOM, 2012). However, around 60% of veterans do not use VA health care services (GAO, 2011b). For example, FY 2010 provided health care to only 5.2 million veterans out of 22 million living veterans (GAO, 2011b). Eligibility is based on veteran status, service-related disabilities, income level, and other factors, and even within the groups eligible for VA care, other factors, such as their proximity to VA facilities and the cost-sharing requirements, might affect the likelihood that they seek care in the VA system (Panangala, 2010).

## Vet Centers

The 300 community-based Vet Centers are located in all 50 states, the District of Columbia, and U.S. territories (IOM, 2012). Vet Centers provide confidential and free counseling, readjustment, and outreach services to all veterans who served in any war zone, to address mental health issues. Vet Centers are often the first point of contact within the VA for veterans and their families, which can help veterans overcome barriers to accessing mental health care. During FY 2010, 191,508 veterans and family members received mental health services (e.g., IOM, 2012).

## VA Mental Health Care Utilization

Whenever analyzing VA mental health statistics, it's important to keep in mind that nearly 60% of veterans do not receive care through the VA (e.g., IOM, 2012). According to a 2011 GAO report on VA health care, during FY 2006 through FY 2010, about 2.1 million veterans received VA mental health care services (GAO, 2011b). Each year the number of veterans receiving mental health care increases, from 900,000 in 2006 to 1.2 million in FY 2010 (GAO, 2011b). OEF/OIF veterans accounted for an increasing proportion of veterans receiving care during this period. In 2010, the VA treated 109,850 OEF/OIF veterans diagnosed with "adjustment reactions," including 96,916 veterans with PTSD; in addition, the VA treated 57,639 veterans diagnosed with depression, 38,715 diagnosed with episodic mood disorders, 45,252 veterans diagnosed with neurotic disorders, and 36,797 OEF/OIF veterans with substance abuse (e.g., GAO, 2011b).

## HOW THE AFFORDABLE CARE ACT AFFECTS MILITARY POPULATIONS

Passage of the ACA raised significant concerns over increased health care costs and reduction of benefits within the military population (Kizer, 2012). Subsequently, efforts have been made by TRICARE, the VA, and even White House officials (see White House, 2012) for public education purposes. In short, according to the VA, the ACA does not impact veterans' eligibility and access to mental health care they might already receive (e.g., VA, 2010), nor does ACA change the TRICARE or TRICARE for Life benefits a family can receive from the VA (e.g., Kizer, 2012). The VA (2010) insisted that veterans enrolled with the VA will not need to obtain additional insurance coverage; however, the ACA will offer veterans an option to enroll in additional insurance plans via new health insurance exchanges that open in 2014. In addition, the VA (2010) reported that veterans with private insurance coverage might benefit from the new ACA consumer protections that prohibit private insurance companies from dropping individuals if they get sick or injured, and veterans will no longer worry about lifetime limits on how much insurance companies will cover in the future.

Most important, under the ACA uninsured veterans and their family members who are currently ineligible for VA or TRICARE mental health care will now be eligible to receive tax credits to purchase insurance via the upcoming exchanges, thus providing access to critical mental health care services (VA, 2010).

## Improved Care for Veterans

According to the GAO (2011b), there are 23.8 million living veterans, but only 7.84 million enrollees in the VA health care system, leaving about 15.96 million veterans not enrolled in the VA health system. Many of these uninsured veterans will have access to quality, affordable health insurance choices through state-based health insurance exchanges, which will foster competition and increase choice, and might be eligible for premium tax credits and cost-sharing reductions as well (Hayley & Kenney, 2012). Therefore, improving the private health care market will help millions of America's veterans as well.

## Preservation of VA Health Care

The ACA states that the VA retains full authority over its health care system in that Congress wrote into the law a provision that VA meets the national standard for health care coverage (VA, 2010). Therefore, there is no foreseeable adverse impact for vets receiving VA mental health care (VA, 2010).

### No required purchase of additional coverage

Because the veterans' health care program meets the standard under the law, veterans enrolled in the VA health care program do not need to obtain additional health care coverage. Veterans may continue to purchase additional coverage if they wish, but the law does not require them to do so (VA, 2010).

### Preservation of TRICARE and TRICARE for life benefits

Similarly, the ACA clarifies that the DoD will maintain sole authority to operate TRICARE by passage of the TRICARE Affirmation Act (H.R. 4887), which lists TRICARE as a government-sponsored program meeting the "minimum essential coverage" requirement (Merlis, 2012). Therefore, there is no anticipated adverse effect on TRICARE or TRICARE for Life beneficiaries (Merlis, 2012). Specifically, TRICARE officials report that there is no provision in the ACA that will lead to increases in copays, changes in eligibility requirements, or in any way modify how TRICARE is administered (TRICARE, 2012a).

### Meeting the individual responsibility requirement

The ACA clarifies that those covered by the VA system and TRICARE for Life meet the individual responsibility requirement via passage of the TRICARE Affirmation Act (H.R. 4887), and therefore exempts TRICARE beneficiaries from penalty (Merlis, 2012; VA, 2010).

## Additional Potential Benefits of the ACA for Military Populations

According to reviews of the ACA's impact on military populations such as an official White House (2012) fact sheet, there are several potential benefits.

### Expanded options for affordable and improved care

The ACA includes provisions to ensure that veterans are provided additional choices for high-quality and affordable care. It allows veterans receiving VA health care to also enroll in an insurance plan through the bill's health insurance exchanges. For middle-income users, the decision about whether to shift from the VA to an exchange plan might again turn on cost-sharing comparisons (White House, 2012). Those with nonservice-connected conditions, and hence paying high VA copayments, could find the exchange plans more favorable (White House, 2012).

### Enhanced flexibility

The ACA will not require changes to current military and veteran's health plans, and at the same time it ensures increased insurance options for military populations, as well as expanded consumer protections to prevent private insurance companies from denying or setting limits on coverage (White House, 2012).

### Insuring uninsured veterans and their families

The most significant benefits of the ACA for military populations is the provision for extending coverage to an estimated 50% of uninsured veterans who would qualify for expanded Medicaid coverage, and an additional 40% who could potentially qualify for government-subsidized coverage through health insurance exchanges, provided they do not have access to affordable employer coverage (Hayley & Kenney, 2012). Of the 40% of the 1.3 million uninsured veterans who served within the last 20 years (and nearly 950,000 of their family members), nearly half are below the age of 45 years (Hayley & Kenney, 2012).

### UNINSURED ADULT CHILDREN

In addition to the concerns over diminished health care benefits for military populations, many are beginning to ask if any of the added benefits associated with the ACA will apply to TRICARE. For example, many beneficiaries with dependent children are asking how the ACA will impact their children aged 26 and younger. Fortunately, this question has already been answered in the National Defense Authorization Act of Fiscal Year 2011 that created the TRICARE Young Adult (TYA) Program, requiring civilian health plans to offer coverage to adult children until age 26, beginning on January 1, 2012.

### EXPANDED COVERAGE FOR VETERANS

Merlis (2012) reported that for potential TRICARE enrollees, the choice to switch to a civilian exchange could depend on whether means-based enrollment fees are enacted. For example, under one proposal, a family of four with income up to $22,589 would pay $680 a year in 2014 (Merlis, 2012). This family is below the federal poverty level for its family size and would qualify for Medicaid at no cost under the ACA. A family with an income of $32,000 in 2014 would pay $920 for TRICARE, whereas that same family would pay about $960 or 3% of family income for subsidized coverage through an exchange plan (Merlis, 2012). All in all, the decision to switch health plans might hinge on whether TRICARE Prime or the exchange offers the lower cost-sharing for military families.

On the other hand, Merlis (2012) opined that TRICARE beneficiaries without access to the Prime network—and hence paying the higher cost-sharing under TRICARE Standard—or those preferring nonnetwork care, might find the exchange plan more appealing. It is unclear at this time which of the mental health services that TRICARE "excludes" might be covered by an exchange.

## UNKNOWN AND POSSIBLE NEGATIVE IMPLICATIONS OF THE ACA ON MILITARY POPULATIONS

Although the ACA offers tremendous promise for improving access and reducing fragmentation for people with mental health or addiction disorders, Kizer (2012) warned that the ACA could also pose a number of unintended negative effects on health care for veterans. For instance, will the existing difficulties in recruiting and retaining qualified mental health staffing in the DoD and VA become exacerbated due to increased access and demand for mental health care by the newly insured, thereby straining the nation's already limited resources? The problem might be averted if current users move to non-VA or TRICARE, but this is uncertain.

Furthermore, the possibility of lower numbers of uninsured people might prompt states and the federal government to cut back on direct (non-Medicaid) financing of mental health care, particularly in light of discretionary spending cuts negotiated as part of the recent debt-ceiling deal (Kizer, 2012). Therefore, military and government leaders might look to dramatically reduce military health care costs by transferring to the civilian sector like the United Kingdom. For instance, British veterans obtain care through the National Health Service (NHS) like everyone else. They have priority when there is a waiting list for services, and there are some programs within the NHS to address veterans' special needs, but there is no separate system (Merlis, 2012). However, it might be easier to make special provisions for veterans in a single-payer system than in one with numerous public and private payers. There are also concerns that civilian providers lack the expertise to identify or treat service-related problems, especially mental health problems. So it seems likely that the VA will have a continuing role.

## NINE PRINCIPLES IN IMPLEMENTING THE ACA THAT COULD TRANSFORM MENTAL HEALTH CARE

Several of the broad goals and provisions of the ACA regarding mental health care bear striking resemblance to those envisioned to transform mental health after World War II and the Korean War. History has taught us that well-intentioned and enlightened policy visions are more frequent than actual programs to improve mental health services within and outside of military health care systems. We offer nine foundational war trauma lessons or "principles" that the ACA appears to at least "touch on" unfinished business of previous war cohorts to overhaul the national mental health system. We examine psychiatric "lessons learned" from the World War II and 21st-century cohort in the form of the 2007 congressionally mandated DoD Task Force on Mental Health (2007), but each are reflected in every war generation's postwar analysis since the 20th century (M. C. Russell & Figley, 2013)

### 1. Elimination of "Medical Dualism" by a Embracing Holistic "Whole Person" Perspective

This first principle focuses on the integration of physical and mental health. The ACA embodies a "whole person" perspective on health and recovery, placing equal emphasis on not only the afflicted individual's physical and mental well-being, but also the importance of familial, sociocultural, morale, and other environmental (e.g., work) factors.

This is evident in part, by the ACA's provisions that focus on parity and the integration of collaborative, culturally sensitive services, as well as by encouraging a continuum of multidisciplinary care coordination including transitions involving work, health, and medical homes (Ofosu, 2011), most of which reflect postwar psychiatric "lessons learned" (Glass, 1966). Stretching the ACA's "whole person" concept further is the single most critical, yet invisible and completely unrealized of all war trauma lessons that was first "learned" (and subsequently forgotten) during the American Civil War (1861–1865) and reverberates as true today, namely, lived embodiment of a holistic view of health and illness—fully equating physical and mental health as inseparable, interdependent components. The unresolved generational debates over the authenticity of war and other traumatic stress injuries, and consequent stigma and disparity between medical and psychological fields, is mainly responsible for the pattern of wartime behavioral crises (M. C. Russell & Figley, 2013). The World War II–era lesson, "When finally, psychiatric casualties were regarded as legitimate consequence of battle stress and strain, it became possible to prepare adequately for their prevention and treatment" (Glass, 1966, p. 22) and "If medical practice is ever to progress to the ideal of psychosomatic medicine, it will require the reorientation of medical training and of all practitioners so that equal emphasis is placed upon the roles of the psyche and of the soma in all illness" (Menninger, 1948, p. 163), mobilized post–World War II efforts to eliminate dualism. In contrast to the endeavors of the Surgeon General in planning for the medical and surgical problems of mobilization, there was no comparable effort in the sphere of military psychiatry (Glass, 1966, pp. 17–18).

A cultural paradigmatic shift toward "holistic health," and clearly eliminating antiquated dualistic beliefs that artificially impart greater value and meaning to bodily aspects of health, will not only incorporate a fundamental war trauma lesson, but it would propel the country's health care system into catching up with 21st-century science, as well as end cyclic wartime crises directly affecting both military and nonmilitary populations. Lessons of war trauma also clearly indicate that resolute "top-down" commitment, organizational structure, and policies reflecting the "whole person" paradigm with equally transparent policy of zero tolerance for perpetuating dualism, stigma, and disparity, is absolutely paramount to effectively meet mental health and social needs of beneficiaries. All other principles listed next are contingent on this first foundational lesson.

## 2. Emphasizing Prevention and Resilience

The second principle is prevention, reflecting critical ACA provisions that address essential changes required to focus more attention and resources on maintaining health and resiliency to reduce cost. Here, too, another key lesson of war trauma is interjected, whereby every modern war generation cites failure to fully implement proven preventative lessons in their postwar analyses (Jones, 1995). For instance, post–World War II "lessons learned" include "In seeking the many causes of psychiatric disability in order to correct them, we must put first the absence of prewar planning to prevent and to treat them. This blunder was made by the War Department and the technical service of the Medical Department, and was ignored by the profession of psychiatry" (Chief of Staff, Gen. Eisenhower, cited in Menninger, 1948, p. 532). However, in the 21st century, continuity of failure to learn this lesson is rampant:

> The mental health needs of service members and family members can only be met by a DOD community that has received adequate training in building resilience and recognizing, responding to, and following up on distress and illness. Unfortunately, DOD's current training related to psychological health is insufficient and inconsistent both across and within the military services. Too little training is evaluated for effectiveness (DoD Task Force on Mental Health, 2007, p. 18).

The ACA appears to give equal importance to mental and social aspects of well-being and illness, with the physical and medical side. If fully realized, the ACA requires multidisciplinary health care teams be staffed with well-trained professionals to address the psychosocial implications of acute and chronic illnesses (Ofosu, 2011). These multidisciplinary teams will practice across the continuum of care, including community and public health clinics, general hospitals, nursing homes, home health care, primary care, hospices, and military and veteran service networks (Ofosu, 2011). However, the greatest obstacle in effectively managing wartime stress casualties has been an inherently fragmented and disjointed military health care system that continues to embrace medical dualism, stigma, and disparity toward mental health. Therefore, the biggest hurdle for implementing the ACA's prevention programs will be how well the nation addresses the first principle.

## 3. Eliminating Mental Health Disparity, Stigma, and Barriers to Care

The third principle of the ACA, and a major unlearned war trauma lesson with fatal implications, is opening access to mental health services by reducing antiquated mental health stigma and disparity between mental and physical health care that constitute harmful barriers to care. The importance of eliminating stigma and disparity is summarized: "In the military, stigma represents a critical failure of the community that prevents service members and their families from getting the help they need just when they may need it most. Further, stigma is of particular concern in the military because of the degree to which military members may bear responsibility for lives beyond their own" (DoD Task Force on Mental Health, 2007, p. 15), harkening back to the World War II cohort. There was a tendency to stigmatize the neuropsychiatric patient as being a failure. When the cause was not physical, then the individual was variously regarded as perverse, subversive, unwilling, weak, or dumb. He was likely to be labeled as a "quitter," "an eight-ball," a "gold brick," or "any of numerous other vernacular disparaging terms" (Menninger, 1948, pp. 20–21), and "When one combines this state of affairs with a prevailing ignorance of and prejudice against psychiatry, it is not surprising that there was a staggering number of psychiatric casualties" (Menninger, 1948, p. 516). However, this lesson, too, was ignored by the 21st-century military: "Evidence of stigma in the military is overwhelming. Of even greater concern are recent findings that service members who screened positive for symptoms consistent with mental illness were twice as likely as those without symptoms to express concerns about stigma" (DoD Task Force on Mental Health, 2007, p. 15), directly contributing to the current wartime crisis. This is astonishing given the robust scientific literature supporting authenticity of stress injuries and justifying a holistic paradigm (IOM, 2008).

A 2010 report published by the Center for American Progress stated, "The total annual cost of racial and ethnic health disparities, including direct medical costs and indirect costs such as lost productivity, lost wages, absenteeism, family leave, and premature death, is of the order of $415 billion" (cited in L. Russell, 2010, p. 2). The ACA addresses well-documented racial and economic disparities by improving access to prevention services in combination with better management and treatment coordination; it is an investment that pays off with better health outcomes and more productive lives at lower cost (Ofosu, 2011). In terms of the broader disparity issue between mental health and medical care, the ACA goes beyond the requirements of the federal parity law by mandating both Medicaid benchmark plans (i.e., alternative plan options created under the Deficit Reduction Act of 2005) and plans to operate via state-based insurance exchanges covering behavioral health services as part of an essential benefits package (Ofosu, 2011). Eliminating differential treatment of mental and medical aspects of care will serve to eradicate any harmful stigma and disparity that will help prevent future wartime behavioral health crises.

## 4. Adequate Supply of Well-Trained Specialists and Quality of Mental Health Services

The most frequently cited and routinely violated war trauma lesson by every generation since the 20th century is the failure to ensure an adequate supply of well-trained specialists who can provide high-quality services across the continuum of care (M. C. Russell & Figley, 2013). For instance, World War II leaders observed, "The importance of assigning well-trained psychiatrists to the divisions cannot be overemphasized. Divisions having such men assigned consistently exhibited a lower neuropsychiatric incidence and a higher return to duty rate than those in which medical officers without such training were arbitrarily assigned as psychiatrists" (Glass, 1966, p. 331); however, "As has been indicated, by the time it was recognized that modern warfare produced a flood of neuropsychiatric casualties, the breach between requirements for psychiatrists and available supply was so great that it was never closed. By the spring of 1945, the shortages and mal-distribution created severe staffing inequities" (Menninger, 1966, pp. 46–47). Tragically, this foundational lesson in meeting wartime mental health needs has been ignored by every subsequent generation, resulting in predictable behavioral health crises as the 21st-century military cohort relearned: "The Task Force arrived at a single finding underpinning all others: The Military Health System lacks the fiscal resources and the fully-trained personnel to fulfill its mission to support psychological health in peacetime or fulfill the enhanced requirements imposed during times of conflict" (DoD Task Force on Mental Health, 2007, p. ES-2), with identical disastrous consequences.

If properly implemented, the ACA holds promise to reverse the harmful trend by containing educational and training provisions to strengthen the mental health care workforce by addressing the education and training needs of clinicians. Workforce development programs in mental health and behavioral health education will assist graduate students specializing in, and providing services to, special high-needs populations such as children, older adults, underserved minorities, and veterans (Ofosu, 2011).

## 5. Early Identification and Intervention

The importance of early identification and intervention in preventing costly chronic disability was widely recognized in World War II: "A most pronounced characteristic of the cases seen early in their illness is the profusion with which new symptoms appear and disappear. As time goes on, without treatment, a more stabilized syndrome crystallizes" (Grinker & Spiegel, 1943, pp. 7–8).

The ACA revised Section 1915(i) of the Deficit Reduction Act of 2005 broadens the home and community-based services waiver option by allowing states to offer benefits specifically intended for people with mental illness and substance abuse disorders and to make care accessible to more people. The section eliminated the requirement that clients meet eligibility for institutional care, thus authorizing earlier interventions for eligible clients (Barry & Huskamp, 2011).

The ACA's emphasis on early identification and intervention resembles another unrealized war trauma lesson:

> Ensuring an easily-accessible full continuum of evidence-based care guarantees effective help is available when most needed. All efforts to

dispel stigma are reduced to hollow promises if, when service members or family members reach the critical juncture where they recognize they need help, they encounter delays, bureaucratic roadblocks or frustration in accessing the services their often complex situation requires (DoD Task Force on Mental Health, 2007, p. 24).

This key lesson was widely reaffirmed during World War II, but it was neglected by 21st-century war planners: "Adequate training of all concerned in the recognition of PTSD and other psychological problems. The Policy Guidance correctly stresses that 'early identification and treatment are key . . .' and that 'medical readiness is a shared responsibility of military commanders, military medical personnel, and individual service members'" (DoD Task Force on Mental Health, 2007, p. 24). As detailed in earlier sections of this report, the current training of commanders and active duty members on recognition and intervention is uneven and generally inadequate. Training of key medical personnel at the smallest unit level, such as medics and corpsmen, is also inadequate (DoD Task Force on Mental Health, 2007).

## 6. Collaborative and Integrative Continuum of Care

The need for coordinating management of serious chronic conditions and comorbidities and "seamless" transitions between various types of services is a central organizing theme in the ACA, as well as a well-documented, but entirely unrealized war trauma lesson. For example, during the 21st century, "Ensuring an easily-accessible full continuum of evidence-based care guarantees effective help is available when most needed" (DoD Task Force on Mental Health, 2007, p. 16). Despite the lessons from World War II, problems in this critical domain remain unaddressed: "There is too little collaboration among the military services to create training material, resulting in wasted time, money, and expertise" (DoD Task Force on Mental Health, 2007, p. 19). Further:

> No single mental health program exists across DOD: Numerous programs related to psychological health are administered within and outside the confines of the Defense Health Program (DHP), with considerable variation in mental health service delivery . . . While the multiplicity of programs, policies, and funding streams provides many points of access to support for psychological health, they may also lead to confusion about benefits and services, fragmented delivery of care, and gaps in service provision (DoD Task Force on Mental Health, 2007, p. 11).

One of the most promising features of the ACA is reducing fragmentation of policies and service delivery by improving the coordination and integration of current programs and newly mandated services (Barry & Huskamp, 2011). The intended level of collaborative, integrated continuum of community-based care is exemplified by the ACA's provision of substance abuse treatment. For instance, in the ACA, substance abuse evaluation and treatment must be incorporated into the central tasks of monitoring and managing medications and educating clients about medication and illness (Ofosu, 2011). This is one of the most challenging areas of behavioral treatment, requiring a mix of integrated services that includes assertive case management; psychoeducation, or a combination of therapy and family-centered education; supported employment; social learning; social support; and harm-prevention orientation. For example, Substance Abuse and Mental Health Services Administration block grants, state-funded behavioral health programs, and initiatives supported by the Medicare-Medicaid Coordination Office, will be made available to design new integrated approaches. Collaborative care makes seamless service provision more feasible, prevents service gaps and client dropout, and avoids duplication and inconsistencies in medication and other treatments.

Section 2703 of the ACA encourages state Medicaid programs to offer a health home option, which is supported by a federal funding match of 90% for the first 2 years. Under this option, states can reimburse a patient-designated health home provider who provides care management, makes necessary referrals, provides individual and family support as needed, and uses health information technology to monitor and coordinate the various service providers involved. Health homes designed for people with severe mental illnesses make it possible for community health centers and other appropriate behavioral health agencies to manage the integration of services over the full range of needs, even when a variety of providers and agencies are involved.

## 7. Ready Access to High-Quality, Definitive, "Whole Person" Care

A fundamental, yet regularly unlearned war trauma lesson relates to "treatability" of stress injuries, especially early:

> Ensuring an easily-accessible full continuum of evidence-based care guarantees effective help is available when most needed. All efforts to dispel stigma are reduced to hollow promises if, when service members or family members reach the critical juncture where they recognize they need help, they encounter delays, bureaucratic roadblocks or frustration in accessing the services their often complex situation requires (DoD Task Force on Mental Health, 2007, p. 24).

This foundational lesson was relearned during the World War II era, but it was ignored and relearned again in the 21st century:

> Easy accessibility of evidence-based best practices for treatment of mental disorders including PTSD. The Policy Guidance stresses these are

treatable conditions, especially early in their progression, and that successful treatment is key to the health of the service member and the mission capability of the force. As noted throughout this report, current resources devoted to providing such treatment are inadequate (DoD Task Force on Mental Health, 2007, p. 24).

The ACA might address these negative trends that have also been replicated in private-sector studies of the quality of mental health and substance abuse treatment finding poor continuity and coordination of care and limited use of evidence-based medical, social, and rehabilitative interventions resulting in costly and inefficient patterns of care (Mechanic, 2012). Payment reform incorporates new forms of adjusted capitation and the related use of bundled or episode payments encourage continuity and efficiency (Mechanic, 2012). By extending the concepts of treatment and related supportive care to such entities as health homes, the ACA provides new pathways for incorporating evidence-based treatments, such as supported employment, that are commonly neglected (Mechanic, 2012).

## 8. Centralized, Comprehensive, and Transparent Monitoring

The DoD should routinely track and analyze patient outcomes to ensure treatment efficacy. The DoD should expedite development of an electronic record that facilitates the systematic collection and analysis of data on the processes and outcomes of care. The Task Force is unaware of any large-scale data collection efforts that assess awareness of the potential for mental health conditions among members of the Armed Forces. Based on information gathered during site visits, there is widespread awareness of the possibility of combat stress or PTSD, and to a lesser extent, TBI. Awareness of other mental health conditions is much more limited.

Section 5.1.1 (Dispel Stigma) and 5.1.3 (Embed Training about Psychological Health throughout Military Life) contain findings and recommendations to raise awareness of mental health conditions. Problems arose in determining the frequency of psychiatric casualties owing to difficulties in obtaining valid comparable neuropsychiatric rates of battle units because somatic complaints were widespread in military personnel during World War II. Despite increasing acceptance of psychiatric casualties, bodily symptoms were regarded as more legitimate reasons for failure to cope with combat or other wartime situational stress. As a result, numerous combat personnel were medically evacuated with various ill-defined organic diagnoses based on somatic symptomatology. Thus there occurred persistent syndromes of headache, digestive upset, low back pain, painful joints, weakness with palpitation, and the like. Most of these complaints represented the usual physical and emotional discomforts of combat participants (Glass, 1966, pp. 996–997). From all this, we could conclude that statistics regarding neuropsychiatric disorders of war will have little significance. The percentage incidences, the proportion of various clinical syndromes, the frequency of predisposing causes, and certainly the recovery rate will be set forth with such a high degree of inaccuracy as to make them of little value. The ACA incorporates several quality measurement initiatives including the reporting of quality indicators on public websites; pay-for-performance programs for hospitals and providers; and organizations' efforts to develop, test, and select high-quality measures (Pincus, Spaeth-Rubless, & Watkins, 2011). A pivotal, routinely neglected war trauma lesson is the need for centralized, comprehensive, and transparent reporting of war stress injuries. During the crucial mobilization and early war periods, however, the lack of planning, preparation, and direction resulted in inadequate or faulty psychiatric policies and practices, wastage of psychiatric personnel, and consequent huge losses of military manpower (Glass, 1966).

The World War II experience clearly indicates the necessity for psychiatric leadership at the highest level of military medicine (Glass, 1966). Certain factors within the Army—its organizations and system—further added to the difficulty for psychiatry. Each of these contributed directly to the production of psychiatric casualties. All of this could be changed so that they would be much less of a menace to mental health.

## 9. Effective Social Reintegration and Community-Support

A critical, albeit universally neglected war trauma lesson is the need to adequately plan and support military populations during transitions, especially social reintegration after leaving military service. This paramount lesson was learned in World War II as reflected by President Roosevelt's December 4, 1944 executive order to his Secretary of War due to high-level concerns of more than 600,000 mostly untreated neuropsychiatric discharged veterans struggling to reintegrate into an unprepared American society:

> My Dear Mr. Secretary:
>
> I am deeply concerned over the physical and emotional condition of disabled men returning from the war. I feel, as I know you do, that the ultimate ought to be done for them to return them as useful citizens—useful not only to themselves but to the community.
>
> I wish you would issue instructions to the effect that it should be the responsibility of the military authorities to insure that no overseas casualty is discharged from the armed forces until he has received the maximum benefits of hospitalization and convalescent facilities which must include physical and psychological rehabilitation, vocational guidance, prevocational training, and resocialization.
>
> Very sincerely yours,
>
> Franklin Delano Roosevelt (cited in Brill, 1966, p. 291)

The World War II–era lesson was repeated in the Army's official "lessons learned" report:

> Rehabilitation, which has as its objective the retraining of individuals to overcome the handicaps of disabilities, the development of self-reliance, and social adjustment and placement in useful work assignment, is largely the responsibility of other government agencies. The medical department of the Army can undertake the beginnings of such rehabilitation simultaneously with medical and surgical treatments (Quinn, 1966, p. 689).

It was also acknowledged by the 21st-century military cohort:

> Continuity of care is essential across all transitions. Military service requires many transitions, including relocation from one base to another. ...Other transitions occur in the context of deployments. ...Another significant and complex transition involves members of the National Guard or Reserve who regularly transition between their military and civilian lives. Finally, the decision to separate or retire from the military is an especially significant transition point for service members and their families (DoD Task Force on Mental Health, 2007, pp. 28–29).

However, knowledge of what is needed and right does not always translate into action, as contemporary military leaders demonstrated by neglecting this essential war lesson.

Several ACA provisions deal with establishing effective community-based social reintegration programs for individuals with chronic, severe medical and mental health conditions, homelessness, substance abuse treatment completers, and prisoners, all facing issues of employment, housing, and health care during social reintegration.

Another benefit of the ACA is supported employment programs that encourage the most severely disabled clients to pursue competitive employment—in other words, employment in jobs that pay at least minimum wage and that are open to anyone in the community—by providing them with support for an unlimited period of time (Mechanic, 2012).

Addressing the risk of homelessness and victimization and providing stable housing are critical to the effective long-term management of serious mental illness. There are a large number of programs to prevent or reduce homelessness, and seven different federal agencies administer such programs. Many homelessness programs are authorized by federal legislation designed to assist the homeless and are available to people in varying circumstances. These programs can be coordinated with other needed behavioral health services, and the various provisions of the ACA present an important opportunity do so to prevent homelessness and incarceration of people with mental illnesses.

## CONCLUSION

Every one of the aforementioned potential changes to the U.S. mental health care system has direct and significant implications for greatly improving the health of military populations, particularly those returning from war and their families. If all of these had been in place prior to the 2001 start of the Afghanistan war, it would have altered the course of the current military mental health crisis.

> It is highly probable that in future wars there will be a similar neglect, in as much as psychiatric disorders are an unpopular and vexing phenomenon. Moreover, the issue of emotional disorders is too readily obscured or confused by moral condemnation and widespread use of such terms as *misfits, cowards,* and *slackers,* all of which make it easy to ignore the problem, particularly when there are so many pressing wartime logistic, training, and personnel requirements (Glass, 1966, p. 738).

If these transformations are implemented within and outside of the military, society can finally be satisfied that we have upheld our pledge to care for the warrior class, and end the shameful cycle of neglect and crisis.

## REFERENCES

Appel, J. W., & Beebe, G. W. (1946). Preventive psychiatry. *Journal of the American Medical Association, 131*, 182–189.

Baker, R. R., & Pickren, W. E. (2007). *Psychology and the Department of Veterans Affairs: A historical analysis of training, research, practice, and advocacy.* Washington, DC: American Psychological Association.

Barry, C. L., & Huskamp, H. A. (2011). Moving beyond parity—Mental health and addiction care under the ACA. *The New England Journal of Medicine, 365*, 973–975.

Best, R. A. (2007). *Military medical care: Questions and answers.* Washington, DC: Congressional Research Service, Report for Congress.

Brill, N. Q. (1966). Hospitalization and disposition. In A. J. Glass & R. J. Bernucci (Eds.), *Medical Department United States Army: Neuropsychiatry in World War II. Vol. I: Zone of interior* (pp. 195–253). Washington, DC: Office of the Surgeon General, Department of the Army.

Cabaj, R. P. (2011). The council on advocacy and government relations. *The American Journal of Psychiatry, 168*, 219–220.

Congressional Budget Office. (2007). *The health care system for veterans: An interim report.* Washington, DC: Congress of the United States.

Congressional Budget Office. (2012). *Updated estimates for the insurance coverage provisions of the Affordable Care Act.* Washington, DC: Congress of the United States.

Defense Manpower Data Center. (2010, April). *Distribution of active-duty and reserve services by service, rank, sex, race report*. Retrieved from www.dmdc.osd.mil/Rank_Gender_Race.xls

Department of Defense Task Force on Mental Health. (2007). *An achievable vision: Report of the Department of Defense Task Force on Mental Health*. Falls Church, VA: Defense Health Board.

Glass, A. J. (1966). Lessons learned. In A. J. Glass & R. J. Bernucci (Eds.), *Medical department United States Army: Neuropsychiatry in World War II. Vol. I: Zone of interior* (pp. 735–759). Washington, DC: Office of the Surgeon General, Department of the Army.

Glass, A. J., & Bernucci, R. J. (1966). *Medical department United States Army: Neuropsychiatry in World War II. Vol. I: Zone of interior*. Washington, DC: Office of the Surgeon General, Department of the Army.

Government Accountability Office. (2011a). *DOD and VA health care—Action needed to strengthen integration across care coordination and case management programs*. Washington, DC: Author.

Government Accountability Office. (2011b). *VA mental health: Number of veterans receiving care, barriers faced, and effort to increase access* (Rep. No. GAO 12–12). Washington, DC: Author.

Grinker, R. R., & Spiegel, J. P. (1943). *War neuroses in North Africa: The Tunisian campaign (January–May 1943). Restricted report prepared for the Air Surgeon, Army Air Forces*. New York, NY: Josiah Macy, Jr. Foundation.

Grob, G. N., & Goldman, H. H. (2006). *The dilemma of federal mental health policy: Radical reform or incremental change?*. New Brunswick, NJ: Rutgers University Press.

Hayley, J., & Kenney, G. M. (2012). *Uninsured veterans and family members: Who are they and where do they live? Timely analysis of immediate health policy issues*. Washington, DC: Urban Institute. Retrieved from www.rwjf.org/content/dam/farm/reports/2012/rwjf73036

Institute of Medicine. (2010). *Provision of mental health counseling services under TRICARE*. Washington, DC: National Academies Press.

Jaffe, S. (2012). U.S. Supreme Court makes historic health ruling. *The Lancet, 380*(9836), 14.

Jones, F. D. (1995). Psychiatric lessons of war. In F. D. Jones, L. R. Sparacino, V. L. Wilcox, J. M. Rothberg, & J. W. Stokes (Eds.), *Textbook of military medicine: War psychiatry* (pp. 1–34). Washington, DC: Borden Institute.

Kizer, K. W. (2012). Veterans and the Affordable Care Act. *Journal of the American Medical Association, 307*, 789–790.

Maze, R. (2009, August 11). Lawmakers: Health care reform won't affect vets' programs. *Air Force Times*. Retrieved from http://host91.242.54.159.gannett.com/benefits/health/military_healthcare_vets_benefits_081109w/

Mechanic, D. (2012). Seizing opportunities under the Affordable Care Act for transforming the mental and behavioral health system. *Health Affairs, 31*, 376–382. doi:10.1377/hlthaff.2011.0623

Menninger, W. C. (1948). *Reactions to combat: Psychiatry in a troubled world*. New York, NY: Macmillan.

Menninger, W. C. (1966). Education and training. In A. J. Glass & R. J. Bernucci (Eds.), *Medical Department United States Army: Neuropsychiatry in World*

*War II. Vol. I: Zone of interior* (pp. 53–66). Washington, DC: Office of the Surgeon General, Department of the Army.

Merlis, M. (2012). *The future of health care for military personnel and veterans.* Washington, DC: AcademyHealth. Retrieved from http://www.academyhealth. org/files/publications/AHMilitaryVetBrief2012.pdf

Military Health System. (2012). *MHS 2012 stakeholders' report: The MHS healthcare to health.* Retrieved from http://www.health.mil/Libraries/Documents_Word_ PDF_PPT_etc/2012_MHS_Stakeholders_Report-120207.pdf

Mojtabi, R., Rosenheck, R., Wyatt, R. J., & Susser, E. (2003). Transition to VA out-patient mental health service among severely mentally ill patients discharged from the armed services. *Psychiatric Services, 54*, 383–388.

Office of Personnel Management. (2009). *Federal employee health benefits program.* Washington, DC: U.S. Office of Personnel Management. Retrieved from http:// www.opm.gov/healthcare-insurance/healthcare/reference-materials/#url=FEHB-Handbook

Office of the Under Secretary of Defense, Personnel, and Readiness. (2006). *Population representation in the military services fiscal year 2006 report.* Retrieved from http://prhome.defense.gov/RFM/MPP/Accession%20policy/ PopRep_FY06

Ofosu, A. (2011). Implication of health care reform. *Health & Social Work, 36*, 229–230.

Panangala, S. V. (2010). *Veterans medical care: FY2010 appropriations (Rep. No. 7–5700, R40737 for Congress).* Washington, DC: Congressional Research Service.

Patient Protection and Affordable Care Act, Pub. L. No. 111–148, 124 Stat. 1025 (2010).

Pincus, H. A., Spaeth-Rubless, B., & Watkins, K. E. (2011). The case for measuring quality in mental health and substance abuse care. *Health Affairs, 30*, 730–736.

Quinn, E. F. (1966). Reconditioning of psychiatric patients. In R. S. Anderson, A. J. Glass, & R. J. Bernucci (Eds.), *Medical Department United States Army: Neuropsychiatry in World War II. Vol. I: Zone of interior* (pp. 687–699). Washington, DC: Office of the Surgeon General, Department of the Army.

Russell, L. (2010, December). *Easing the burden: Using health care reform to address rural and ethnic disparities in health care for the chronically ill.* Washington, DC: Center for American Progress.

Russell, M. C., & Figley, C. R. (2013). *Generational wartime behavioral health crises: Part one of a preliminary analysis.* Manuscript submitted for publication.

TRICARE. (2012a). *Evaluation of the TRICARE program: Access, cost, and quality, fiscal year 2012 report to Congress.* Falls Church, VA: TRICARE Management Activity (TMA)/Office of the Chief Financial Officer (OCFO)—Defense Health Cost Assessment and Program Evaluation (DHCAPE), in the Office of the Assistant Secretary of Defense (Health Affairs) (OASD/HA). Retrieved from http:// www.tricare.mil/hpae/_docs/TRICARE2012_02_28v5.pdf

TRICARE. (2012b). *TRICARE behavioral health care services: TRICARE behavioral health care services are available for you and your family.* Falls Church, VA: TRICARE Management Activity. Retrieved from http://www.tricare.mil/mybenefit/ Download/Forms/BHC_FS.pdf

U.S. Census Bureau. (2010). *A snapshot of our nation's veterans*. Washington, DC: Author. Retrieved from http://www.census.gov/how/infographics/veterans.html

U.S. Census Bureau. (2012). *American Community Survey: Response rates—Data*. Washington, DC: U.S. Census Bureau. Retrieved from http://www.census.gov/acs/www/methodology/response_rates_data/index.php

U.S. General Accounting Office (GAO). (2003). *Report to congressional committees: Military personal: DOD needs more data to address financial and health care issues affecting reservists*. (Publication no. GAO-13-1004). Washington, DC: Author.

U.S. Government Accountability Office. (2006). *Defence health care: Access to care for Beneficiaries who have not enrolled in TRICARE's managed care option* (GAO-07-48). Washington, DC: Author.

Veterans Administration. (2010, June). *VA health care information for veterans about health care reform*. Washington, DC: Author. Retrieved from http://www.visn20.med.va.gov/docs/HealthCareReformFactSheet1614.pdf

White House. (2012). *Health reform for American veterans and military personnel*. Retrieved from http://www.whitehouse.gov/sites/default/files/rss_viewer/health_reform_for_veterans.pdf

# Index

Note: Page numbers followed by 'f' refer to figures, followed by 'n' refer to notes and followed by 't' refer to tables.

**Numbers**

1915 (c) HCBS waivers 99, 103

**A**

accountable care organizations (ACOs) 17, 91–2, 94, 126–7

*Action for Mental Health* 165

ADS Center (Resource Center to Promote Acceptance, Dignity and Social Inclusion Associated with Mental Health) 80

adult children 1, 90, 112, 158; TRICARE Young Adult (TYA) Program 182

adults without children 37, 112

Adverse Childhood Experiences (ACE) Study 11, 156, 157

Aetna project 69–70t

Agency for Healthcare Research and Quality (AHRQ) 62–5, 76–7

Akin, Todd 127

alternative benefit plans (ABPs) 37, 38

Americans with Disabilities Act (ADA) 2008 98, 101, 130, 132

**B**

Barnes, J. 78

barriers: to implementing *Olmstead* plans 105–6; to integration 76–8, 77t; war trauma lessons for ACA principle of eliminating 185–6; to women's care 124–6

behavioral health and intellectual/ developmental disability county and city programs: next steps for 95; population and service implications for 93–4; staffing implications 94–5

behavioral health consumers and families, ACA for: electronic health record (EHR) technology 114; elimination of limits on coverage 112; essential health benefits 111–12; federally qualified health centers (FQHCs) 113–14; health homes 113; health insurance expansion 110–11; home and community based services 115–16; parity for mental health and substance abuse services 113; Planning and Advisory Councils (PACs) 116–21; preventative services 115; recovery model 114–16; shared decision making (SDM) 114–15; substance abuse services 113; telemedicine 114

behavioral health disorders, gradual move into mainstream: and ACA 14–17, 34–7; Bush's New Freedom Commission 9–12; changing clinical perceptions 11; Clinton health reform 7–9; consequences of failure to fully fund services for 9–10; denial of medical care 5; "dual diagnosis" 13; health insurance limits on 6, 31, 33; inability to find health insurance 5; innovations moving forward 17–18; parity, campaign to achieve 6–7, 13–14; preventable health problems 12–13; separate systems 5–6; spotlight on mental health 8–9; and trauma 11–12

bidirectional integration 49

brain research 12

Buck, J.A. 40, 113–14

Bush, President George W. 9, 14

business model, levels of integration 59t

**C**

California Endowment 81

cancellation, policy 166

cancer app 134–5

*Capitol People First et al. v. CA Dept of Developmental Services et al.* 104

# INDEX

care management 34, 39, 41, 77, 77t; programs for mental health 64, 66, 67t, 69t, 70t
caregiving burden 128–30; ACA addressing 130
catastrophic cap 176
catchment areas 47
Center for American Progress report 2010 186
Center for Integrated Health Solutions (CIHS) 53–4, 61
Center for Medicare and Medicaid Services (CMS) 37, 99, 100, 116
*Chambers et al. v. City of San Francisco* 104–5
children and adolescents under ACA 79, 126
clinical delivery, levels of integration 58t
Clinton, President Bill, health reform 7–8, 8–9
collaborative care: definitions 51–2t; model 49, 62; three-level model 50; war trauma lessons for ACA principle of 188–9 *see also* integrated care
Colorado Access project 68–9t
community-based services: *Olmstead* ruling on 98 *see also* Medicaid home- and community-based services
Community First Choice Option 106
community health planning 47–8
Comprehensive Health Planning and Public Health Services Act 1966 47
consumer advocacy group, Maryland 21–30; background to mental health advocacy 22–3; behavioral health integration 23–4; federal parity implementation 24; health reform following ACA 23–4; seven Cs of effective advocacy 25–30
consumers, behavioral health *see* behavioral health consumers and families, ACA for
contraceptives 124, 125, 127
copayments: elimination 90, 124; VA mental health 171
county and city behavioral health and intellectual/developmental disability programs: next steps for 95; population and service implications for 93–4; staffing implications 94–5
coverage, insurance: deductibles and copays 90, 124; expansion 110–11; family coverage to age 26 1, 90, 112, 158, 182; gaps in mental health and substance abuse 39–41, 40f; individual mandates 35, 36; limits to behavioral health 90, 112, 166, 180; long-term care cover 39; noncoverage for mental health and substance abuse disorders 32; preexisting

condition exclusions 90, 125–6; reform, ACA 90
Criminal Justice/Mental Health Consensus Project 10–11
criminal justice system intersecting with mental health systems 10–11
culturally and linguistically appropriate services 79, 140, 157

## D

deductibles, elimination of 90, 124
Deficit Reduction Act (DRA) 2005 100, 186, 187
DeGruy 78
demographics, changing 140–4, 141f, 142f, 143t
depression 65; and diabetes 68t; integrated care and effects on 63–4
diabetes, IMPACT mental health projects 67–8t
discrimination, insurance companies: against ethnic minorities 47, 49; against women 126, 131
DoD Task Force on Mental Health 177, 183, 185, 186, 187, 188, 189, 190, 192
Domenici, Senator Pete 7
domestic violence 132–3
Downtown Emergency Service Center (DESC) 1811 Program 76t

## E

Eagleville Hospital 47
early identification and intervention 123, 157; war trauma lessons for ACA principle of 187–8, 189–90
educational attainment 146, 147t
electronic health record (EHR) technology 77–8, 92–3, 114
Employee Retirement Income Security Act of 1974 (ERISA) 7
employer-sponsored health insurance 32, 33
employment programs, ACA supported 192
enrollment process 121, 157–8, 159; PAC involvement 119–20
essential health benefit (EHB) requirements 35–6, 53, 111–12; choosing state benchmarks for 36, 46, 89–90, 112; incorporation of MHPAEA 38
*Essential Health Benefits Bulletin 2011* 16
ethnic minorities: caregiving burden 128–9; discrimination against 47, 79; integrated care and effects on depression 63; and stigma of mental illness 79–80; using technology to address health disparities 134 *see also* racial and ethnic

# INDEX

communities, impact of ACA on behavioral health care

evidence-based practices 133–4, 190; addressing health equity and health disparities 155–7; collaborative care model 49, 62; mental health and primary care levels of integration 56t

**F**

Families USA 120, 124

family coverage to age 26 1, 90, 112, 158; TRICARE Young Adult (TYA) Program 182

Federal Committee on the Costs of Medical Care 46

Federal Employee Health Benefits Program (FEHBP) 169

federal funding: block grants 40, 114, 117, 118, 189; for comprehensive health planning 48; to develop EHRs 93; to extend HCBS programs 100; for Medicaid expansion 36, 37, 39, 89

federally qualified health centers (FQHCs) 92, 113–14

financial barriers to integration of primary and mental health care 77, 77t, 78

Fluke, Sandra 124

four-quadrant clinical integration model 53, 54, 54f, 61

funders committed to ACA 80–1

**G**

gaps in insurance cover 39–41, 40f

good standing 35

Grand Junction, CO integrated care study 78

Great Britain 183

**H**

HARP (Health and Recovery Peer) Project 71–2t

*Health Care in a Context of Civil Rights* 47

health care in mental health settings projects: HARP (Health and Recovery Peer) Project 71–2t; VA integrated care clinic 70–1t

health disparities: ACA enrollment and participation to reduce 157–8; Center for American Progress report 2010 186; and health equity in racial and ethnic communities, ACA addressing 139–40, 154–7, 156f; racial and ethnic communities 149t, 151; and social class 88; *Unequal Treatment: Confronting Racial and Ethnic Disparities in Health Care* 139–40; using technology to address 134; war trauma lessons for ACA principle of eliminating 185–6

health homes 45, 53, 62, 91–2, 94, 113, 126–7, 189

health insurance exchanges 35, 89–90, 111, 158; Pacific Island Jurisdictions, Puerto Rico and US Virgin Islands 144–5; population and service implications for county and city programs 93–4; veterans and option to shift from VA to 181, 182

Health Insurance Portability and Accountability Act (HIPAA) 1996 78

health plan mental health integration projects 68–70t; Aetna 69–70t; Colorado Access 68–9t

health service planning 47–8

*Health Services Integration: Lessons for the 1980s* 46–7

holistic approach to health care: ACA support for 53, 115, 139; need for ready access to 189–90; women with disabilities 133–4; World War II and lessons learned 164, 183–4, 189–90

home and community based services *see* Medicaid home- and community-based services

home health benefit, mandatory 98–9

homelessness 9–10; ACA programs to reduce 192

horizontal integration 49

"Housing First" model 10, 76t

Huber, T. 45, 50, 78

**I**

IMPACT mental health projects: applications to patients with diabetes 67–8t; DIAMOND/Adaptation of IMPACT model 67t; research trials 67t

individual mandates 35, 36

information technologies 92–3, 95

institutionalization: Medicaid long term bias towards 105, 106; *Olmstead v. L.C. (1999)* Supreme Court ruling on 97–8 *see also Olmstead* litigation study

institutions for mental diseases (IMDs) 5, 6

Integrated Behavioral Health Project, California 63–5

integrated care 44–86; access levels 55t; advantages and weaknesses at each level of collaboration/integration 59–60t; barriers to 76–8, 77t; bidirectional integration 49; bipolar disorder, effects on 64; business case for 62–3, 65–6, 76; business model 59t; characteristics of integration linked to process of care 52, 52f; clinical delivery 58t; cocurring disorders, treatment for 48–9; collaboration and collaborative care

## INDEX

model 49, 61; data levels 56t; definitions 49, 51–2t; depression, effects on 63–4; Downtown Emergency Service Center (DESC) 1811 Program 76t; economic benefits 62–3, 65–6, 76; electronic health record (EHR) technology 77–8; essential health benefit (EHB) categories 53–4; evidence-based practice levels 56t; examples of primary health services interrelating with mental health and SUD services 45–6; financial barriers to 77, 77t, 78; forms of integration 48–9; four-quadrant model 53, 54, 54f, 61; funding levels 55t; governance levels 56t; Grand Junction, CO study 78; health care in mental health settings 70–2t; health homes *see* health homes; health plan mental health integration projects 68–70t; health planning agencies 47–8; historical background 46–8; horizontal integration 49; IMPACT mental health projects 67–8t; Integrated Behavioral Health Project, California 63–5; in Maryland 23–4; mental health/primary care integration model 53, 55–6t; model projects, examples 65, 67–76t; models of integration 53–61; Northern California Kaiser Permanente substance use studies 72–4t; PACs and encouraging 118; panic disorder, effects on 64; patient experience 58t, 66; patient outcome measures 62–5; physical health, effects on 64–5; practice/organization 59t; Primary and Behavioral Health Care Integration (PBHCI) Program 53, 61; Puentes Integrated Medical Care 75–6t; SAMHSA integration programs 61–2; Screening and Brief Intervention (SBI) studies 74–5t; service levels 55t; six levels of collaboration/integration 54, 57–60t, 61; space levels 57t; standard framework for levels of integrated health care 54, 57–60t, 61; stigma of mental illness, addressing 79–80; substance abuse, effects on 64; three-level model of collaborative care 50; underserved populations, implications of ACA integration 78–81; U.S. Preventive Services Task Force (USPSTF) 74t; vertical integration 49; war trauma lessons for ACA principle of 183–4, 188–9; Washington State substance use and medical cost studies 75t; workforce skills 116
intellectual/developmental disability and behavioral health county and city programs: next steps for 95; population

and service implications for 93–4; staffing implications 94–5

### J
Joint Commission on Mental Illness and Health (JCMIH) 164–5

### K
Kennedy, Patrick 14
Kennedy, President John F. 5

### L
language: barriers to health care 79, 140, 157; fluency 146–7, 147t
life expectancies 12, 91, 112
*Ligas et al. v Hamos et al.* 104
limits to behavioral health insurance cover 6, 31, 33; ACA elimination of 90, 112, 166, 180; employer-sponsored insurance 33; MHPAEA 33–4, 39, 113; non-quantitative treatment limits (NQTLs) 34
long-term support and services (LTSS) 40, 40f, 42, 100, 106

### M
managed behavioral health care (MBHC) industry 41
mandatory home health benefit 98–9
Maryland: early adopter of ACA 23 *see also* consumer advocacy group, Maryland
Medicaid: bias towards institutionalization 105, 106; home model 17, 114; institutions for mental diseases (IMDs) excluded from 5, 6; managed care long-term services and supports (MLTSS) programs 40, 40f, 42, 100, 106; performance reform and changes in financing 92, 127; psychiatric illnesses in people enrolled in Medicare and 63, 65
Medicaid expansion 1, 16, 36–7, 78–9, 88–9; alternative benefit plans 37, 38; effect on populations served by county and city programs 93–4; eligibility standards 36, 88, 111; estimated percentages of people with behavioral health conditions enrolling in 88–9; federal funding 36, 37, 39, 89; implications 37; meeting needs of racial and ethnic communities 152–4, 153f, 153t, 154t, 155f; specialized benefit packages 37; a state option 16, 23, 89, 111, 152, 153–4, 153f, 159; Supreme Court ruling 16, 37, 89; in Texas 89
Medicaid home- and community-based services 98–9; 1915 (c) HCBS waivers 99, 103; ACA provisions to expand 106, 115–16; barriers to implementing *Olmstead* plans 105–6; elderly target

## INDEX

group 103; initiatives to expand programs 99–100; mandatory home health benefit 98–9; participants. increase in 100; personal care services (PCS) program 99; Section 1115 Research and Demonstration waivers 100; spending, increase in 100; State Plan benefit 100, 106; waiting lists for 98, 99, 103, 106

Medicare: limits on psychiatric services 6; military and veteran personnel 171, 175; performance reform and changes in financing 92, 127; psychiatric illnesses in people enrolled in Medicaid and 63, 65; and treating women with disabilities 133

Medicare Act 1965 45

Medicare Improvement Act 2008 18n

*Mental Health: A Report of the Surgeon General* 8–9

Mental Health Association of Maryland (MHAMD) 21–30; background to mental health advocacy 22–3; behavioral health integration 23–4; federal parity implementation 24; health reform following ACA 23–4; seven Cs of effective advocacy 25–30

Mental Health Parity Act 1996 7, 13–14

Mental Health Parity and Addiction Equity Act (MHPAEA) 2008 14, 31–2, 113, 165–6; background 32–4; incorporation with EHB 38; insurance and financing issues 39–40, 40f; interaction with ACA 37–40, 39t; key features 33; limits to behavioral health insurance cover 33–4, 39, 113; non-quantitative treatment limits (NQTLs) 34; scope of services issue 34; seen as a threat by MBHC 41

Mental Health Planning and Advisory Councils (PACs) 116–21; education programs 120; encouraging integration of mental health and substance abuse services 118; mandated purposes 117; membership 117; monitoring and evaluating services 118–19; role in enrolling individuals in health insurance plans 119–20; use of new technologies 120; West Virginia Mental Health Planning Council (WVMHPC) 118, 119

mental health/primary care integration model 53, 55–6t

mental health settings, health care in: HARP (Health and Recovery Peer) Project 71–2t; VA integrated care clinic 70–1t

Mental Retardation and Community Mental Health Centers Construction Act 1963 165

military and veteran mental health services: ACA effect on 179–82; active duty component 167; comparative study of insured and uninsured veterans 172–3; differential impacts of ACA 166–73; DoD civilian employees 169; eligible beneficiaries 173–4; family members 171–2; in Great Britain 183; historical context 164–6; improved care for veterans, ACA 180; military retirees 169–70; overview of Department of Veterans Affairs 178–9; potential positive impact of ACA 166; preservation of VA health care, ACA 180–2; reserve component 167–9; transitioning to VA health care system 177–8; uninsured veterans and former military personnel 172–3, 180, 181–2; unknown and possible negative implications of ACA 182–3; veterans and eligibility for VA mental health benefits 170–1

military and veteran mental health services, nine war trauma lessons for implementing ACA: collaborative and integrative continuum of care 188–9; early identification and intervention 187–8; effective social reintegration and community support 191–2; eliminating disparity, stigma and barriers to care 185–6; elimination of "medical dualism" 183–4; emphasizing prevention and resilience 184–5; monitoring of patient outcomes 190–1; ready access to quality "whole person" care 189–90; supply of well-trained specialists and quality of services 186–7

military health care system, overview 173–7; comparison of out-of-pocket expenses for families vs a civilian HMO 177; deficiencies in military mental health care 177; eligible beneficiaries 173–4; estimated costs of mental health care 174; mental health care services 175–6; TRICARE covered mental health services 176; TRICARE health plan costs 176–7; TRICARE health plan options 174–5; TRICARE mental health exclusions 176

Miller 78

monitoring: and evaluating services 118–19; of mental health patient outcomes 190–1

moral hazard 33

## N

National Alliance on Mental Illness (NAMI) 7, 18n, 22, 120

National Association of State Mental Health Program Directors' (NASMHPD) 12, 13, 112

# INDEX

National Family Caregiver Support Program
130
National Institute of Mental Health (NIMH)
164
National Prevention, Health Promotion and
Public Health Council 115
New Freedom Commission on Mental
Health 9–10, 15; goals 19n
Nichols, L. 78
non-quantitative treatment limits (NQTLs)
34
Northern California Kaiser Permanente
substance use studies 66, 72–4t; costs of
family members 73–4t; Integrated Medical
Care 72–3t; role of primary care in 5-year
outcomes 73t; role of psychiatry in 5-year
outcomes 73t
nursing mothers in workplace 126

## O
Obama, President Barack 4, 8, 14, 15, 80
Older American Act 2000 130
*Olmstead* litigation study 97–109; ACA
provisions to address Medicaid's
institutional bias 106, 115–16; barriers to
implementing *Olmstead* plans 105–6;
*Capitol People First et al. v. CA Dept of
Developmental Services et al.* 104; case
outcomes 103–4, 104t; *Chambers et al. v.
City of San Francisco* 104–5; class action
status 102, 104; data analysis 101; data
sources 100–1; delays in litigation process
105; diagnoses of plaintiffs 103, 103f;
discussion 105–6; elderly persons and
103; findings 101–5, 102f, 103f, 104t;
HCBS services 98–9; HCBS services,
expansion 99–100; *Ligas et al. v Hamos et
al.* 104; and "reasonable effort" theory 99;
settlement agreements 104; Supreme
Court ruling 97–8
One Mind Campaign 12

## P
Pacific Island Jurisdictions, Puerto Rico and
US Virgin Islands 144–5, 144f
parity, mental health: campaign for 6–7,
13–14; Mental Health Parity Act 1996 7,
13–14 *see also* Mental Health Parity and
Addiction Equity Act (MHPAEA) 2008
patient: experience, integration 58t, 66;
monitoring of outcomes 190–1; outcome
measures research 62–5
Patient Care and Affordable Care Act of
2010 (ACA): background 14–17;
behavioral health and 34–7; interaction
with MHPAEA 37–40, 39t; major

components 88–93; nine principles for
implementation 183–92; signing into law
4; states and implementation 16–17; U.S.
Supreme Court ruling 16, 37, 89
performance reform, ACA 92
personal care services (PCS) program 99
Planning and Advisory Councils (PACs) *see*
Mental Health Planning and Advisory
Councils (PACs)
poverty, living in 37, 132, 140, 147, 147t,
150t
practice/organization, levels of integration
59t
preexisting conditions: elimination of
exclusions for 90, 125–6; racial and ethnic
communities 158; women 125–6, 131
premiums, health care 35, 90, 157; TRICARE
168, 169, 170, 177; women's 124, 125, 126
preventable health problems, mental illness
and 12–13
preventative care: for mental health services
and substance abuse 115; war trauma
lessons for ACA principle of 184–5;
women's health 124–5
Primary and Behavioral Health Care
Integration (PBHCI) Program 53, 61
primary care settings: barriers when
providing mental health services 78;
improved outcomes for depression
management in 63; preferred by mental
health patients 62; provision of behavioral
health care services 45–6, 95; and
reduction in stigma of mental illness 62,
79–80
prison and jail populations 79, 145–6
private health insurance: expansion and
reform 34–6, 38; subsidies 35, 36
Program of All-Inclusive Care for the Elderly
(PACE) 156–7
Puentes Integrated Medical Care 75–6t
Puerto Rico 144, 144f, 145

## Q
qualified health plans (QHPs) 35
quality: measurement initiatives, ACA 191;
reforms, ACA 91–2

## R
racial and ethnic communities, impact of
ACA on behavioral health care 139–61;
addressing health equity and health
disparities, ACA 139–40, 154–7, 156f;
Adverse Childhood Experiences (ACE)
Study 11, 156, 157; changes in racial and
ethnic makeup of US 140–4, 141f, 142f,
143t; demographic profiles 146–7, 147t;

202

## INDEX

enrollment and participation to reduce health disparities, ACA 157–8, 159; health disparities 149t, 151; leading causes of death 147, 148t; Medicaid expansion 152–4, 153f, 153t, 154t, 155f; mental health conditions 150t, 151; population of Pacific Island Jurisdictions, Puerto Rico and US Virgin Islands 144–5, 144f; prison and jail populations 145–6; Program of All-Inclusive Care for the Elderly (PACE) 156–7; special health issues, risks 148t, 151; substance use disorders 151, 151t
racial discrimination 47, 49
Ramstad, Jim 14
rape 127–8
recovery, focus on 114–16
Reducing Cancer Among Women of Color App Challenge 134–5
Rehabilitation Act 1973 98
reintegration, war trauma lessons for 191–2
Resource Center to Promote Acceptance, Dignity and Social Inclusion Associated with Mental Health (ADS Center) 80
Roosevelt, President Franklin D. 191

### S

SAMHSA (Substance Abuse and Mental Health Services Administration) 61–2, 80, 115, 118
Screening and Brief Intervention (SBI) studies 74–5t
seven Cs of effective advocacy 24–30
sex education programs 126
shared decision making (SDM) 114–15
small group health insurance, expansion and reform 34–6, 38
smoking and tobacco use 13
social justice 88
social reintegration programs 192
standard framework for levels of integrated health care 54, 57–60t, 61
State Balancing Incentive Program 106
State Plan benefit 100, 106
states: ACA implementation 16–17; alternative benefit plans 37; budgets for mental health programs 40; EHB benchmarks 36, 46, 89–90, 112; financial benefits of Medicaid expansion 89; health insurance exchanges, implementation 89; option on Medicaid expansion 16, 23, 89, 111, 152, 153–4, 153f, 159; uninsured populations 89, 152, 153t, 154t, 155
stigma, mental health 9, 12, 62; integrated care addressing 79–80; war trauma lessons for ACA principle of eliminating 185–6

substance abuse: ACA provision for integrated continuum of community-based care 188–9; effects of integrated care on drug use 64; estimated percentages of people under Medicaid expansion suffering disorders 88–9; gaps in coverage for mental health and 39–41, 40f; PACs and issues of 118; potential shortage of service providers 41; preventative services 115; problems in prison and jail 145; racial and ethnic communities 151, 151t; services, review of implications of ACA on 113–14 *see also* substance abuse studies
Substance Abuse and Mental Health Services Administration (SAMHSA) 61–2, 80, 115, 118
substance abuse studies: Downtown Emergency Service Center (DESC) 1811 Program 76t; Northern California Kaiser Permanente 72–4t; Puentes Integrated Medical Care 75–6t; Screening and Brief Intervention (SBI) studies 74–5t; U.S. Preventive Services Task Force (USPSTF) 74t; Washington State substance use and medical cost studies 75t

### T

tax credits 35, 111, 125, 180
tax penalties 35, 36
telemedicine 114
Teva Women's Health survey 124
Texas 89
trauma 11–12, 115 *see also* military and veteran mental health services, nine war trauma lessons for implementing ACA
TRICARE: ACA and preservation of 181; comparison of out-of-pocket expenses with a civilian HMO 177; coverage denied for abortions for rape and incest 128; covered mental health services 176; and deficiencies in military mental health care 177; eligible beneficiaries 173–4; Extra 167, 168, 170, 172, 175; family members cover 171–2; health plan costs 176–7; for Life 175, 181; mental health exclusions 176; military retiree coverage 169, 170; overview 173; Prime 167, 170, 172, 174–5; Retired Reserve (TRR) 168–9; Standard 167, 168, 170, 172, 175; Young Adult (TYA) Program 182
Troutman, Dr Adewale 159
Turning Point Program 48

### U

underserved populations, implications of ACA integration 78–81

# INDEX

*Unequal Treatment: Confronting Racial and Ethnic Disparities in Health Care* 139–40

uninsured population: family coverage to age 26 1, 90, 112, 158, 182; to gain health coverage under ACA 34, 163; impact of ACA and MHPAEA interaction on 38; prior to passage of MHPAEA 32; racial and ethnic minorities 140, 152, 154t, 155, 155f, 156f; by state 89, 152, 153t, 154t, 155; veterans and former military personnel 172–3, 180, 181–2

U.S. Preventive Services Task Force (USPSTF) 74t

U.S. Supreme Court: *Olmstead v. L.C. (1999)* ruling 97–8; ruling on ACA Medicaid expansion 16, 37, 89

## V

Van Egeren, L. 45, 50, 78

vertical integration 49

Vet Centers 179

veteran health services: ACA and preservation of VA health care 180–2; improved health care for veterans, ACA 180; integrated care clinic 70–1t; mental health care utilization 179; overview of Department of Veterans Affairs 178–9; transitioning to VA health care system 177–8; vet centers 179; veteran eligibility for mental health benefits 170–1

Veterans Programs Enhancement Act 1998 178

## W

Washington State substance use and medical cost studies 75t

Weinberg, M. 78

Wellstone, Senator Paul 7

West Virginia Mental Health Planning Council (WVMHPC) 118, 119

White House Conference on Mental Health: 1999 8; 2013 80

W.K. Kellogg Foundation 48

women with disabilities 130–4; comprehensive care for whole woman 133; defining disability 130; empirically supported treatment 133–4; finding and affording health insurance 132; preexisting conditions 131; victimization assessment 132–3

women's health 122–38; ACA key provisions for 79, 124; barriers to preventative care, ACA addressing 124–6; caregiving burden 128–30; contraception and reproductive care 124, 125, 127; and health homes 126–7; health insurance costs 125; nursing mothers in workplace 126; preexisting conditions under ACA 125–6; rape 127–8; Reducing Cancer Among Women of Color App Challenge 134–5; use of technology under ACA 134–5; women with disabilities *see* women with disabilities; workforce issues 135–6

workforce, mental health: staffing implications for county and city programs 94–5; and supporting women's health 135–6; and veterans' health 183; war trauma lessons for 186–7